Caring for People with Challenging Behaviors

Essential Skills and Successful Strategies in Long-Term Care

SECOND EDITION

by

Stephen Weber Long, Ph.D.

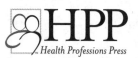
HPP
Health Professions Press

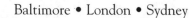
Baltimore • London • Sydney

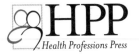

Health Professions Press, Inc.
Post Office Box 10624
Baltimore, Maryland 21285-0624

www.healthpropress.com

Copyright © 2014 by Stephen Weber Long
All rights reserved.

Interior and cover designs by Mindy Dunn.
Typeset by Barton Matheson Willse & Worthington, Baltimore, Maryland.
Manufactured in the United States of America by Versa Press, East Peoria, Illinois.

The case studies in this book are based on the author's experience. They are composite accounts that do not represent the lives of specific individuals, and no implications should be inferred.

The information provided in this book is in no way meant to substitute for the advice or opinion of a medical, legal, or other professional or expert. This book is sold without warranties of any kind, express or implied, and the publisher and author disclaim any liability, loss, or damage caused by the contents of this book.

Library of Congress Cataloging-in-Publication Data

Long, Stephen Weber, author.
    Caring for people with challenging behaviors : essential skills and successful strategies in long-term care / by Stephen Weber Long. — Second edition.
        p. ; cm.
    Includes bibliographical references and index.
    ISBN 978-1-938870-12-5 (paper)
    I. Title.
    [DNLM: 1. Behavioral Symptoms—prevention & control—Case Reports. 2. Caregivers—psychology—Case Reports. 3. Long-Term Care—psychology—Case Reports. 4. Patient Care Planning—Case Reports. 5. Professional-Patient Relations—Case Reports. WM 165]
    RC451.4.N87
    362.16—dc23
                                                                                    2014030722

British Library Cataloguing in Publication data are available from the British Library.

E-book edition: ISBN 978-1-938870-35-4

Contents

DOWNLOADABLE RESOURCES

DOWNLOAD

See **For the Reader** for information on how to use the exercises, handouts, and posters for *Caring for People with Challenging Behaviors*. All handouts and exercises from the chapters, as well as the blank forms in the book appendix, are available for *free* download at www.healthpropress.com/caring-downloadable-resources (use password m2f37rg).

The following posters are available for free download at www.healthpropress.com/caring-downloadable-resources (use password m2f37rg)

Understanding Causes of Challenging Behaviors

Active Listening

Allowing Choices

Using Praise, Compliments, and Acknowledgment

Things to Avoid When Trying to Encourage Positive Behaviors

The ABCs of Behavior

Holding On: Dealing with Reactions to Challenging Behaviors

Realistic Goals for Challenging Behaviors

Cooperative Problem Solving

Either-Or, All-or-Nothing Thinking

Avoiding Physical Harm by a Care Recipient

Common Caregiver Reactions to Care Recipients' Difficult Behavior

Essentials of Care

Re-evaluating Shoulds and Unenforceable Rules

Setting Limits in Relationships

About the Author

Stephen Weber Long, Ph.D., is a psychologist and psychoanalyst. He received a doctoral degree in clinical psychology from the California School of Professional Psychology in Berkeley/Alameda, California, and a postdoctoral diploma in psychoanalysis and psychotherapy from Adelphi University.

Beginning in 1992, Dr. Long was the Extended Care staff psychologist at the Department of Veterans Affairs Medical Center in Northport, New York, for 15 years. As staff psychologist, he served as a trainer to caregiving staff, counselor to patients and residents, and consultant to the medical center's supervisors and administrators. Overlapping with his time in the Extended Care staff psychologist position at the Northport VA, Dr. Long maintained a private psychoanalytic practice, served as the president of the Adelphi Society for Psychoanalysis and Psychotherapy, and was an executive board member of the Postdoctoral Programs in Psychoanalysis and Psychotherapy at Adelphi University's Gordon F. Derner Institute of Advanced Psychological Studies.

Since the publication of the first edition of *Caring for People with Challenging Behaviors: Essential Skills and Successful Strategies in Long-Term Care*, Dr. Long has continued the general practice of psychoanalytic psychotherapy, has provided staff training to extended-care facilities in the United States, and has continued in his role as a consultant to extended-care administrators and supervisors.

Preface to the Second Edition

Writing the first edition of *Caring for People with Challenging Behaviors: Essential Skills and Successful Strategies* was a particularly meaningful experience for me. It helped me to focus my attention on bringing together several interests: the needs of people who require care; the needs of hands-on caregivers; the needs of supervisors and administrators in professional caregiving settings; the work of researchers; and my own experience of working in a long-term care setting for nearly 15 years.

Since the first edition was published in 2005, I have been fortunate to be invited to provide staff training and consultation on the principles and techniques described in the book at a number of long-term care settings in the United States. It has also been rewarding to meet people who have read the book on their own. Those who have attended training sessions and other readers often have pointed out that although the book focuses on long-term care settings, the principles and techniques are also helpful for family caregivers and those working in other professional caregiving settings or programs, such as assisted living facilities or professionally provided home-based care. This second edition has been revised to acknowledge the broader audience for the material in the book and includes material new to this edition. Some of the revised material increases the focus on empowering caregivers to deal with the stress of their roles, while some of the newer material offers further consideration of how to effectively integrate into the culture of long-term care the skills and principles for addressing challenging behaviors.

Although there are aspects of this second edition that were not in the first, the basic approach described in the first edition for dealing with the difficult or challenging behaviors of people who need close attention, care, and assistance remains fundamentally the same. It is an approach to psychological practice that is endorsed by the American Psychological Association (APA), and is what the APA refers to as "evidence-based practice in psychology," that is, practice that integrates the best available research evidence with clinical expertise and the needs and values of the patient or client. It is practice that can include the aim of enhancing public health by applying empirically—scientifically—supported principles of psychological assessment, case formulation, therapeutic relationship, and intervention. The Afterword to this edition is intended for those who may be interested in the theory underlying the principles and techniques in this book.

Finally, a number of readers of the first edition who have expressed that they enjoyed the book have explained that the frequent use of stories about caregivers and care recipients added a level of feeling to the reading that enhanced their understanding of the material. This edition also relies heavily on stories that are examples of caregivers and those to whom they provide care. Although the stories are set in long-term care communities, the principles and techniques they address also apply to care that is provided in the home either by professional caregivers or by family members.

It is my hope that this new edition will continue to serve readers and care recipients alike by providing valuable tools and education for effective responses to challenging behaviors.

Acknowledgments

Many people have influenced the writing of this book. The residents, staff, and administrators of a number of long-term care settings contributed greatly to my understanding of the lives and concerns of care recipients, caregivers, and those who create and administer programs and facilities. Readers of the first edition of *Caring for People with Challenging Behaviors: Essential Skills and Successful Strategies in Long-Term Care* include those who have found it helpful in providing care for family members at home. Their feedback led to the second edition being written in a way that acknowledges that the principles and techniques described in the first edition also apply in their situations.

My friends Judith Ackerhalt, R.N., Ed.D., and Pearl Ketover Prilik, D.S.W., along with all of my colleagues and teachers at Adelphi University's post-doctoral program in psychoanalysis and psychotherapy at the Derner Institute of Advanced Psychological Studies, played a role in inspiring me to write both the first and second editions of this book.

Preparing a book for publication, even updating an existing book to make a second edition, can be an anxiety-provoking experience. However, Mary Magnus and Cecilia González of Health Professions Press were skillful guides in bringing this second edition through the process of publication. It was a true pleasure to work with them.

Finally, as many other authors have noted, those closest to us can have a profound influence on the successful completion of a writing project. I am deeply fortunate and grateful to have my wife, Helen, my daughter, Elaine, and my son, Adam. Whether I needed to laugh, complain, sit and watch TV, or get back to work, they helped me keep these and other parts of my life in balance, sharing in my experience as they let me share in theirs.

Introduction

It is not unusual for people who receive close care, attention, and assistance to behave in challenging, or difficult, ways. In fact, up to 80% of long-term care residents are described as having moderate to severe behavior problems. Such problems are a primary reason for family members deciding to place a loved one in a long-term care setting. Difficult behaviors also happen in other care settings, such as assisted living, and as part of professionally provided home-based care.

Many people who begin working in long-term care settings are surprised by how often they see, experience, or hear about care recipients behaving in difficult ways. It is common for those who need care to resist what others try to do with or for them by insulting or threatening others, yelling, shouting, or screaming. Although less common, there are also instances when a care recipient hits, scratches, kicks, or even bites. Challenging behaviors are frequently aimed at caregivers.

Family caregivers are sometimes not surprised by the difficult behaviors of a family member who is in need of care. They may describe the behaviors as "just the way he (or she) has always been." Sometimes, however, difficult behaviors or actions may be dramatic changes and are very upsetting to caregivers.

Caring for People with Challenging Behaviors: Essential Skills and Successful Strategies in Long-Term Care is intended as a guide for professional and family caregivers. Its aim is to help reduce or eliminate many typical behavior challenges of care recipients. In this book, the term *challenging behavior* refers to any behavior that causes emotional or physical harm to either the person engaging in the behavior or to someone else. From this point of view, hostile behavior aimed at someone else is a challenging behavior. If a behavior hurts someone unintentionally, it is still considered a challenging behavior. In addition, behaviors related to depression, anxiety, or fear can be considered challenging behaviors. This book details techniques for successfully addressing such behaviors.

An environment that supports the use of these techniques can increase how helpful they can be. In long-term care facilities and professionally provided home-based care programs the effectiveness of these skills is strengthened when staff, supervisors, physicians, and administrators, as well as family members, have a common understanding of the skills and their importance. When family members or significant others are primary caregivers in the home, the effectiveness of the techniques will be increased if family members in general understand and support their use. Whether you are an administrator, a supervisor, a professional hands-on caregiver; whether you are a student or a veteran in the field of long-term care; whether you are caring for a spouse, a parent, a grandparent, or another significant person in your life, this book is meant for you.

Dealing with challenging behaviors is often stressful to caregivers, and learning ways of reducing or eliminating stress is very important in empowering us to provide successful care. Throughout this book you will find detailed descriptions of methods of managing stress that many people find effective.

Caring for People with Challenging Behaviors can also assist mental health professionals who provide consultation to families and administrators and staff of long-term care settings and programs on how best to approach a difficult situation with a particular person being cared for. The principles and skills outlined in this book also can be used to create workable treatment plans that address common troubling behaviors.

This book can be a valuable part of training programs as well. It may be used as a basis for in-service training of staff, supervisors, and administrators. It may also be used as part of the overall training of those who are preparing to begin work in long-term care settings or programs. In addition, it may be used in classes or workshops for family caregivers.

Often when someone in need of care behaves in a troubling way, the behavior is related to an illness, such as Alzheimer's disease. Challenging behaviors are also sometimes related to other conditions that are more often thought of as mental illnesses, such as depression or schizophrenia. Physical pain or discomfort can also influence a person to behave in difficult ways. Sometimes a challenging behavior is related to lifelong attitudes, habits, or personality. The methods described in this book are appropriate for use with individuals whose behavior is affected by any of these influences.

Whenever a mental or physical illness seems to be contributing to a care recipient's challenging behavior, it is important to seek the advice of appropriately qualified healthcare professionals. Even in cases when a mental or physical illness is not clearly involved, it is important to consult with trained and experienced healthcare or mental healthcare professionals if a challenging behavior is persistent. *Caring for People with Challenging Behaviors* is not intended to replace the advice of physicians, nurse practitioners, social works, psychologists, or any appropriately trained or experienced professionals. Yet, it is important that the skills described in this book be a central part of treating the problem, regardless of cause. They really are skills for all of those who help, whether day-to-day staff, medical specialists, administrative staff, family members, or other significant people, in the life of someone who requires care.

Chapter 1 discusses why people in need of care do the things they do. The chapter looks at major influences on behavior through specific examples of how physical functioning, thinking, feeling, the way some behavior seems to lead to other behavior, and interactions with others can affect what someone does. Chapter 1 ends with a discussion of coping with stress. It also describes the importance of increasing the number of pleasant events that can be enjoyed each day as one approach for caregivers to manage stress.

Chapter 2 offers examples of ways to encourage a care recipient's positive behaviors. The chapter is based primarily on three ideas: 1) the more a behavior is reinforced, the more it will occur; 2) the more a positive behavior is reinforced, the less often a difficult behavior will happen; 3) a care recipient's experience of interactions with others can be the most important source of reinforcing positive behaviors. This chapter describes the steps of active listening, a communication skill for developing an empathic, emotional understanding. Such listening and understanding reinforces many positive behaviors, as it encourages a care recipient to value his or her relationship with caregivers. Other ways of encouraging positive behaviors are explored as well, such as allowing people who are dependent on care to make choices and praising, complimenting, or acknowledging positive behaviors. The chapter ends by discussing the stress management technique of progressive muscle relaxation.

Chapter 3 is about problem solving. It describes a way of looking at a situation, particularly interpersonal interactions (or "relationship situations"), to understand what might trigger or reinforce a challenging behavior. Knowledge of possible triggers and reinforcers can be used to help the care recipient reduce or eliminate the behavior. The chapter also describes a two-step process for helping reduce frequent demanding or attention-seeking behaviors. Chapter 3 contains several examples of how to use problem-solving steps to work with individuals to help them eliminate or reduce challenging behaviors. Chapter 3 also explains the importance of "holding on," or containing, our reactions to difficult behavior. Finally, mental imagery is explored as a stress management technique for caregivers.

The main point of Chapter 4 is to look more deeply at dealing with stress related to the difficult behavior of those to whom we provide close care, attention, and assistance. The chapter examines how our thinking and feeling can be affected by those whose behavior is challenging and how our own thinking habits can cause or add to our stress. This chapter is about exerting conscious influence on our own thoughts and feelings in order to feel less stressed by the challenging behavior of those who depend on our care. How we deal with such stress directly influences how effectively we address challenging behaviors. In addition, Chapter 4 considers how our feelings about those whose behavior is difficult and the things they do can help us in understanding and responding. The chapter concludes by describing a breathing-focused technique for deepening relaxation and stress management.

In Chapter 5 we look at the use of behavior (or behavioral) contracts and advance directives, both of which may be used in addressing challenging behaviors. This chapter and its contents are completely new to the second edition. The focus is on some limitations of the use of behavior contracts and on the potential benefits of using advance directives for mental health, behavioral health, and stress management issues related to challenging behaviors. Behavior contracts and advance directives may be of most interest to those working in long-term care facilities or programs. Family members of those who are long-term care residents or clients, or of those who may become residents or clients, may also find the discussion of behavior contracts and advance directives helpful. Chapter 5 also describes steps for how caregivers can use forgiveness as a way of managing stress reactions to the difficult behavior of others. This part of the chapter may be useful to every reader in some way.

Chapter 6 examines factors that can interfere with the effective use of the techniques described in this book, including our own personal obstacles to effectively using the techniques, the environment of a long-term care facility or program, and societal attitudes toward aging and illness. The chapter provides ways of addressing these different obstacles and encourages us to see ourselves, long-term care settings and programs, and society as parts of a system—what we do affects the other parts of the system and can promote positive change. Chapter 6 ends by considering the importance of good relationships in managing stress and offers ways to improve relationships.

Chapter 7 is a guide to treatment planning for addressing challenging behaviors. The chapter presents a five-step treatment plan guide for individual caregivers. Although the guide for individual caregivers is presented in a format for professional caregivers, it can also be used by individual family caregivers at home. Chapter 7 includes another five-step treatment plan guide for professional treatment teams. In addition, this chapter describes how to integrate educational material based on *Caring for People with Challenging Behaviors* into the day-to-day routine of a facility, an approach aimed at increasing and deepening all staff members' familiarity with effective techniques for addressing challenging behaviors. The goal of this approach is also the *prevention* of many behavior problems, because prevention is the best possible treatment. Finally, Chapter 7 can be a useful tool for mental health professionals called on for consultations in cases involving the challenging behaviors of those in need of close care, attention, and assistance.

For the Reader

Skillful use of the techniques described in *Caring for People with Challenging Behaviors: Essential Skills and Successful Strategies in Long-Term Care* takes practice. These approaches can often be described in simple language. Mastering them, however, is an ongoing process that involves using the techniques in various situations with various people. Descriptions of the techniques are supplemented with exercises that are gathered at the end of the chapters and are intended to help readers develop or deepen their mastery of needed skills. The exercises can be useful both for those who use the book independently or as part of in-service or classroom education. They can enhance readers' familiarity with the skills by encouraging active thinking about how they can be used. In addition, the exercises may help start or expand classroom discussion.

Helping staff, management, administrators, and family members remain familiar with—and deepen their familiarity with—the psychological principles and techniques addressed in this book can be an important part of taking a preventive approach to the behavior problems of those dependent on our care. Even when behavior problems are not a focus of formal treatment planning, however, it is important to promote the use and understanding of these techniques and principles in ways that become a part of a caregiving culture. Making discussion and awareness of the material addressed in this book routine can promote such a culture.

Use of the Handouts and Posters

In long-term care facilities, advancing discussion and awareness can involve materials such as the poster series for *Caring for People with Challenging Behaviors* (available for download from Health Professions Press with the purchase of this book [www.healthpropress.com/caring-downloadable-resources (use password m2f37rg)]). The posters can be displayed on a rotating basis, with copies of the first poster hanging in appropriate locations for approximately 4 weeks, copies of the next poster appearing for approximately 4 weeks, and so on. Good places to hang them include staff break rooms and conference rooms—anywhere staff, treatment planning team members, supervisors, and members of the administration meet.

The posters correspond to some of the book's handouts, which can be photocopied and distributed. (The handouts are also available for download from Health Professions Press with the purchase of this book [www.healthpropress.com/caring-downloadable-resources (use the password m2f37rg)].) See Chapter 7 for more information about handout topics.) As soon as a poster is presented, copies of the accompanying handout can be distributed to all staff members (including clerical, housekeeping, and food service staff), treatment planning team members, supervisors, and administrators. Immediate supervisors can distribute the handouts. For example, charge nurses on different shifts can give handouts to the nursing staff members on their shifts. The facilitator of treatment planning team meetings or another designated person can distribute the handouts to team members present at the meetings. This person also can ensure that members of the administration receive copies.

Supervisors can briefly discuss each handout with staff. Treatment planning team meeting facilitators can do this with the team. Review and discussion of each handout can be added to the agenda of regular meetings attended by members of the long-term care facility administration as well.

The person who coordinates staff education in the facility or another designated person can ensure that posters are rotated and that corresponding handouts are given to supervisors and meeting facilitators. This coordinator may design quizzes with one or two true-or-false questions based on each handout. Anyone who would like education credits that count toward the facility's requirements can complete the quizzes. Completed quizzes on four posters might be considered verification of an hour of continuing education.

Although it may be most helpful to display only one poster during each 4-week period, some posters immediately before or after another poster in the series may contain closely related information. In such cases, you might choose to display two to four posters at the same time. In this situation, the handouts that correspond to these posters would be distributed for review and discussion as well.

Using the procedures outlined here, the series of posters and handouts can cycle through each year. This process can be an important part of a long-term care facility's efforts to meet the educational needs of personnel and the psychological needs of residents.

Dedicated to
Michael, Victor, Karen, Laura, Ellen, and Tina.

You are always with me.

Why People Who Need Care Do What They Do

A number of things influence the behavior of someone who needs care. When we are interested in reducing or eliminating common troubling, or challenging, behaviors, it can be helpful to keep these influences in mind. This chapter looks at some of the major influences on how people in need of care behave. This chapter also points out that it is important to deal effectively with the stress that we are under in order to deal effectively with the challenging behaviors of those in need of care. A method for increasing the pleasant things that we do for ourselves is described at the end of the chapter. It is one way of coping with stress.

Internal and External Influences on Behavior

One way to look at causes of challenging behavior is to think about what internal and external things might be triggering the behavior. Typically, a challenging behavior—that is, a behavior that is harmful physically or emotionally—happens because of internal *and* external factors. In fact, it is often hard to say whether a challenging, or difficult, behavior is either completely internal or external. Every challenging behavior is likely to be triggered or reinforced by both internal and external things. For example, a person may have vision trouble and difficulty making decisions because of impaired brain functioning. These might be considered internal challenges. This person may act confused and irritable in dim or low lighting or when moving from a well-lit area to a dark area. In this case, the light-ing could be an external cause of the individual's behavior. If caregivers cannot understand the combination of internal and external influences, they are not able to provide aid effectively (by correcting the lighting, for example). In ways like this, what caregivers do or do not do can also become an external influence on the person's behavior. See Handout 1.1 and the sections that follow in this chapter for more information. In addition, try completing Exercise 1.1.

Physical Functioning

Physical functioning refers to how a person's body works (for example, how well a resident's muscles and joints move or how well he or she breathes). Physical func-tioning also means how different areas of the brain work, particularly the areas that play an important part in a person's ability to pay attention, remember new things, control emotions, think clearly, talk, understand others, and tell what is and is not real.

The physical functioning of a person who needs close attention and care can influence how he or she behaves. Someone with severe arthritis may avoid moving parts of the body that hurt. Someone who has great difficulty breathing may avoid doing things that could make it harder to breathe. An individual who is increasingly unable to remember new or recent events may talk only about the past. Another person who believes things are happening that others cannot see or hear may behave in ways that are unusual and seemingly unpredictable. The cases that follow illustrate how various physical issues can affect an individual's behavior.

Mrs. Wells

Mrs. Wells was 92 years old. The pain of the severe arthritis in her hips made it difficult for her to walk, stand, or sit. Even lying in bed in one position for long periods was painful. Before she entered a long-term care residence, Mrs. Wells spent most of each day in bed to avoid further pain. Because this kept her from doing much, she lost a good deal of her overall muscle strength. Mrs. Wells be-came so frail that when she fell on the way to the bathroom one day at home, she broke her hip. She continued to stay in bed during her time in the long-term care residence.

In Mrs. Wells' case, the physical condition of arthritis influenced what she did. To avoid further pain, she stayed in bed.

Ms. Quigley

Ms. Quigley was 77 years old. Over a number of years her ability to breathe de-clined. Using medications for breathing and oxygen helped, but she still gasped for breath even when she walked only a few steps. Ms. Quigley breathed more easily when she sat in a chair beside her bed, so that is what she did most of the day.

Mr. D'Angelo

Mr. D'Angelo was 83 years old. He had what seemed to be Alzheimer's disease. His illness, a type of dementia, interfered with his brain's ability to function well. He could, however, carry on a pretty good conversation. Mr. D'Angelo particularly liked talking about baseball and the major league teams of his childhood and early adulthood. He also liked to watch baseball games on television. He wondered, however, about some of the teams that he saw playing. Mr. D'Angelo said that he had never heard of many of them, and that he did not know who any of the players were either.

Mr. D'Angelo was not able to remember recent events because of how his dementia affected his brain's functioning. One effect on his behavior was that he mostly talked about the distant past. In addition, he usually did not follow through on things that he had agreed to do, such as going to the dining room when told it was mealtime, because he often forgot about agreeing to do anything.

Mr. Siegler

Mr. Siegler was 70 years old. For most of his adult life, he had a serious mental illness. His illness significantly affected his ability to see reality as most other people do. At times, he thought that things existed or happened that no one else saw or believed. Mr. Siegler occasionally told staff members in his long-term care community that he was tired of being spied on. He said that the reason he sometimes stood motionless and quiet in his room—and the reason he often did not respond to people talking to him—was because there were microphones all over his room. The microphones, he explained, were taping every sound, and the tapes would be used against him. Mr. Siegler's mental illness contributed to his extremely guarded behavior.

Emotions

It is not easy to define the word *emotion*, yet most of us know an emotion when we feel one or see one in another person. We usually recognize happiness, sadness, love, and anger as emotions. Emotions are feelings, a combination of parts of us that are often thought of as mental and physical. Our emotions influence and are influenced by our experience of ourselves and the world around us. A person who needs care can feel happy or unhappy about certain events that happen in the world. While someone receiving long-term care who has a tendency to feel happy may be more likely to take an optimistic view of events, another person receiving long-term care who tends to feel unhappy may be more likely to have a negative view.

Emotions can have a strong influence on what someone in need of care does—that is, how he or she behaves. One who often feels embarrassment or shame might avoid others. Another who typically feels lonely might frequently look to others for company. Feeling frustrated, annoyed, or angry could make someone in need of care more likely to argue with or insult others. A person who is fearful of others may shun social interaction whenever possible. Building on the previously presented cases, the cases that follow show effects of emotion on behavior.

Mrs. Wells

Mrs. Wells said that she usually stayed in bed to avoid the pain of the arthritis in her hips. However, she also described feeling depressed. She could not understand why she was depressed. God had granted her a long, full life, she said. It made no sense to her that after receiving such a gift she would feel so miserable. Mrs. Wells felt sinful and guilty because she thought her depression meant that she was ungrateful for all that God had given her. Feeling guilty made her feel more miserable, which then made her feel more guilty. She was afraid other people would see how bad—how sinful—she was. Feeling ashamed, she did not want other people to see her. This cycle deepened Mrs. Wells' depression.

Mrs. Wells' emotional experience of depression contributed to her isolation. She avoided having visitors, sometimes by telling anyone who came to see her that she was just too tired for a visit. The way that Mrs. Wells acted was very much influenced by her emotions.

Ms. Quigley

For Ms. Quigley, just getting out of bed to sit in the chair at her bedside made it hard for her to catch her breath. She also felt nervous nearly all of the time. Ms. Quigley knew that the medications she took to help her breathe had the side effect of making her feel nervous. She also said that she had been a nervous person her whole life.

Beyond the side effect of her medication, Ms. Quigley said she did not know what made her nervous. She noted that her anxiety worsened when she was alone. She hated being alone, and she hated feeling anxious. As a result, Ms. Quigley often called for help, even for things that she was able to do on her own. At times, she acknowledged that when she felt lonely she also felt more like she needed help.

Ms. Quigley's emotional experience of anxiety often motivated her to seek help, even with tasks she was able to do on her own. Getting attention this way apparently protected her from feeling more alone and anxious.

Mr. D'Angelo

Mr. D'Angelo's dementia made it hard for him to remember new information. Eventually, he had difficulty concentrating or paying attention. He was easily distracted from any task in which he was involved. When he started getting dressed in the mornings, he sometimes left his room while he was not fully dressed. When a nursing assistant helped him get dressed, Mr. D'Angelo would show signs of frustration and annoyance at having to focus on tasks such as putting his socks on, putting his arms through his shirt sleeves, and getting his shirt buttoned. His frustration, annoyance, and growing anger led him to insult whoever was involved in helping him dress. Sometimes these insults were aimed at the other person's race or gender.

Mr. D'Angelo's dementia caused changes that could make him frustrated. In turn, his anger periodically had an unpleasant effect on his behavior.

Mr. Siegler

Part of Mr. Siegler's mental illness was that he often felt very afraid. In fact, his strongest and most persistent feeling seemed to be fear. He said his fear came from the threat posed by people "we all know" but about whom it was not safe to say anything more specific. He believed that they were collecting evidence against him to punish him in some unspeakable way.

For Mr. Siegler, the strength of his fear significantly contributed to his withdrawn and guarded behavior. He rarely spoke to or interacted with others.

Thinking

Thinking is often considered a kind of self-talk. Frequently it is described as what we tell ourselves, usually silently in our own minds. Self-talk can be about many topics: ourselves, others, our experience of the world around us, and our beliefs.

How a person receiving care thinks can have a major influence on how that person behaves. For example, if the person thinks that he or she is bad and feels guilty, that individual might tend toward isolation to avoid having others see this badness. Another person who considers being alone a terrible thing may often try to get the attention of others and keep them from leaving. If a person who requires close care and attention thinks that other people are always trying to control what he or she does, that person may act uncooperatively or combatively, struggling to maintain, or regain, a sense of his or her own control. Yet another person might think that others would disapprove of his or her thoughts and feelings. If this individual expects punishment from others because of these thoughts and feelings, he or she might try to avoid situations that would reveal them. The cases that follow further show ways in which thinking can affect behavior.

Mrs. Wells

In her depression, Mrs. Wells tended to think of herself as a bad and sinful person. She thought that if other people were with her, they would see how bad and sinful she was. Mrs. Wells avoided others to avoid being treated as she believed she deserved—with cruelty and neglect.

How Mrs. Wells thought about herself affected the way she acted and contributed to her self-imposed isolation.

Ms. Quigley

Ms. Quigley was filled with anxiety when she was alone. While alone, she kept thinking that something terrible was going to happen and that no one would be there to help her. As a result, Ms. Quigley tried to think of ways to make people come to her so she would not be alone.

Even when people were with Ms. Quigley, she continuously thought about when they would leave her. She thought of how unbearable being alone would be. As a result, Ms. Quigley created ways to make people stay with her.

These thoughts contributed to Ms. Quigley's frequently asking for, or insisting on getting, help with tasks that she could do independently.

Mr. D'Angelo

Mr. D'Angelo often said that other people were trying to make him do what they wanted him to do. He thought people wanted him to stop doing what he preferred and to start doing something else. Occasionally, he said he knew that he was not thinking clearly and often did not make the best decisions. He said he was losing himself, the person he had always experienced himself to be, and losing control over what was happening to him.

Mr. D'Angelo's thoughts apparently influenced him to act uncooperatively as a way of asserting his sense of self. His thoughts seemed to move him to resist feeling that his dwindling sense of himself was being overwhelmed. These thoughts appeared to increase the likelihood of Mr. D'Angelo's verbal attacks on staff members at his long-term care residence, people who saw themselves as only trying to help him. To Mr. D'Angelo's way of thinking, however, he was not attacking them; he was defending himself.

Mr. Siegler

Mr. Siegler thought that if others knew what he was thinking and feeling, they would attack him. Mr. Siegler tried to keep anything he did or said from showing what he thought or felt to avoid being reprimanded, attacked, or punished. Mr. Siegler's thinking contributed to his acting in ways that isolated him from others. Only rarely was he able to let his guard down enough with anyone to say how fearful he was and how he expected to be abused.

Behavior Influencing Further Behavior

Behavior is frequently thought of as action that can be seen or observed by others. Walking, talking, sitting, eating, laughing, and crying are all examples of behavior.

Our own behavior influences what we do next. For example, if a person takes a long walk, that might trigger him or her to sit down. In a long-term care situation, the behavior of someone who needs care can have an impact on what he or she does. One who is withdrawn and stays in bed may express a decreasing interest in getting out of bed. While the person remains in bed, he or she will not have experiences that could trigger and reinforce behaviors other than staying in bed. For this resident, staying in bed would contribute to an increased amount of time spent in bed. A resident who engages in few self-care activities may call for help frequently. A person who resists the help of caregivers may spend more time performing tasks independently. Another person who rarely speaks to others may continue to spend most of his or her time in solitude. The cases that follow present examples of behavior further influencing behavior.

Mrs. Wells

As noted, Mrs. Wells stayed in bed not only because of her arthritis pain, but also because she wanted to avoid having visitors. By behaving in this way, Mrs. Wells was severely limiting her possibilities of experiencing the everyday, pleasant events that could have reduced or eliminated her depression and its negative impact on her overall physical and mental health. For example, by staying in bed, Mrs. Wells did not see sunsets. She was not able to see children playing, birds flitting about in the trees, people walking by, or slow-moving clouds against a blue sky. The possible positive effects on her emotional life and general health of experiencing everyday positive events were lost to Mrs. Wells as she remained in bed.

Ms. Quigley

It seemed that the less Ms. Quigley did for herself, the more she called for help. Ms. Quigley's helpless behavior appeared to diminish her independence and contribute to her help-seeking behavior.

Mr. D'Angelo

For a while, when Mr. D'Angelo resisted what staff members tried to do with him, he said things such as, "I don't need any help!" or "Don't I have any say in what is going on around here!" He would frequently insist that he could do things on his own and make his own decisions. When he was asked why he so frequently clashed with staff, Mr. D'Angelo said it was the only way to keep from being taken over. As his dementia progressed, Mr. D'Angelo's ability to use words and think clearly decreased. He became more likely to resist staff physically, by pulling away, hitting, or kicking.

When Mr. D'Angelo was verbally or physically combative, this behavior seemed to escalate. His resisting behavior seemed to contribute to further resisting behavior.

Mr. Siegler

Mr. Siegler behaved in ways that isolated him from others. He stayed to himself and rarely said anything to anyone. As a result, the things he thought about— such as being spied on or being abused for what he thought or felt—could not be changed by comparing his experience with what others actually said or did. Engaging in isolating behavior contributed to Mr. Siegler's continued isolating behavior.

Interactions with Other People

During interactions, what one person does or says influences what others do or say. In other words, what people do affects what other people do.

The behavior of people in need of care is often influenced by their experience of the behavior of the people around them. For example, a person in need of close care and attention who is told "don't talk that way" when speaking of feeling despair may, under certain circumstances, withdraw from social interaction. This may be most true if the person feels despair most of the time. The resident may interpret "don't talk that way" as an admonition that the greater part of his or her current experience of life is not acceptable.

Another resident who often calls for assistance and is told not to call so much may react by calling more often. This particularly can be the case if, for example, the resident feels helplessly alone and fears that those who say not to call so much will leave the resident alone more often. Feeling more loneliness and fear, the resident's calling for help might increase.

A caregiver will often help someone in need of care with activities such as showering, getting dressed, eating, standing, or getting into bed. Sometimes the person in need of care will react to this help with anger. Although the angry reaction may seem unprovoked, it is important to recognize that the response happened during an interaction. Despite a caregiver's, or staff member's, best intentions, there will be times when a care recipient, or resident, experiences an interaction differently than the other person expects or thinks makes sense. Uncooperative, combative, threatening, and withdrawing behaviors are likely to be influenced by interactions between or among people. To fully understand these behaviors in a way that can help to reduce or eliminate them, we need to work to understand how the person in need of care experiences the interactions that influence difficult behaviors. The cases that follow are examples of this principle.

Mrs. Wells

Mrs. Wells' daughter visited her at least once a week. A common scenario follows:

Mrs. Wells said that she was too tired for a visit, and her daughter replied, "You can't be tired, Mother. You're in bed all the time, even though you shouldn't be." When Mrs. Wells said that she felt miserable, her daughter stated, "You just have to stop wallowing in self-pity, Mother. Stop thinking about everything being wrong." Then, when Mrs. Wells became tearful and cried, her daughter said, "Mother, please stop; I can't bear to see you cry."

Mrs. Wells felt worse—that is, more depressed—during and after these visits than before. She believed that her daughter could not tolerate her, that her daughter was reacting to her being bad and doing, thinking, and feeling the wrong things: being in bed was wrong, thinking about her problems was wrong, and crying was wrong.

Mrs. Wells' experience of interactions with her daughter reinforced her feelings of being alone in how she felt, of hopelessness, and of being a bad person. It reinforced her desire to avoid people so she could avoid their reaction to how bad and how sinful she was. It reinforced her behaving in ways aimed at keeping to herself.

Ms. Quigley

Jen, a nursing assistant new to the long-term care community, was assigned to work with Ms. Quigley. Each day for a week, Jen hurried to Ms. Quigley's room whenever she used the call bell or cried out for help. Ms. Quigley called often for help with, for example, finding her glasses when they were on the table next to her or knowing what kind of soup was on the lunch tray in front of her.

It was impossible for Jen to help all of the other residents assigned to her and do everything else she needed to do while constantly running to Ms. Quigley. She spoke with her supervisor, who asked the attending physician, Dr. Pasignine, to speak to Ms. Quigley about her attention-seeking behavior.

Dr. Pasignine explained to Ms. Quigley that the staff wanted to help her with whatever she needed, but that she had to realize that she was not the only person for whom the staff members offered care. The doctor asked Ms. Quigley to call only when she really needed help.

Ms. Quigley said that she did only call when she needed help. She said that nobody seemed to understand just how sick she was and how much help she needed. They did not realize, she explained, that when she was left on her own she was frightened about how much she needed someone to help her. As Ms. Quigley spoke, her breathing became shallower and quicker. After Dr. Pasignine told her that staff members would do their best to ensure that she got the care she needed, Ms. Quigley's breathing improved. Unfortunately, following the doctor's visit, Ms. Quigley called for help even more often than she had before.

When a staff member asked about her increasing calls for help, Ms. Quigley explained that, following Dr. Pasignine's visit, she felt even more anxious and fearful. She said that maybe Dr. Pasignine would do what she could for her, but that the doctor often was not available. Ms. Quigley said that she only felt more certain that no one would come to her when she really needed help. Apparently, Ms. Quigley's experience of her interaction with Dr. Pasignine had a significant impact on her subsequent behavior.

Mr. D'Angelo

Tara, a nursing assistant, went to Mr. D'Angelo's room to help him dress. At first he said, "Okay," and was pleasant with Tara when she said she was going to help him get dressed. As Tara was getting clothes from the dresser, she asked Mr. D'Angelo to get out of bed. He did not respond, and the following interaction took place:

Tara went to the bed and tried to coax Mr. D'Angelo to sit up by taking his hand and saying, "Okay, here we go."

Mr. D'Angelo pulled his hand away and cried, "What are you doing?"

"Mr. D'Angelo, it's time for you to get up," Tara responded.

"What are you talking about? I'm not getting up," Mr. D'Angelo said crossly.

Tara said, "Mr. D'Angelo, you can't stay in bed all day. The doctor said it's not good for you to be in bed all day."

"Oh, the doctor said that?" Mr. D'Angelo said.

Tara continued, "That's right. So here, let me help you sit up." Tara held out her hand to Mr. D'Angelo.

"What do you want now?" Mr. D'Angelo asked impatiently.

Because things were not going well, Tara decided to let Mr. D'Angelo stay where he was. She decided to help him get ready for the day a little later.

Mr. D'Angelo's lack of cooperation was not unusual. In the past, he was more likely to argue, complain, or insult others as he resisted help. Gradually, though, he resisted by not responding to requests, pulling away, and making brief statements or questions, such as, "What are you doing?" This change in the way he resisted seemed to show that his dementia was progressing and affecting the parts of his brain involved in the more complicated thinking required to express arguments or complaints. The dementia's progression also appeared to make it more difficult for him to remember things that were said or done just minutes earlier. At this point, resisting or fussing seemed to be the only ways for him to express what he had previously expressed in words. Mr. D'Angelo struggled to retain some measure of control. He seemed to experience his interaction with Tara as another instance of having no say in what was happening to him.

Mr. Siegler

Ben, a new recreation therapist in the long-term care community, found Mr. Siegler in his usual spot—his room. Ben said hello, introduced himself, and told Mr. Siegler which therapeutic recreational events were coming up that day. When Mr. Siegler did not respond, Ben asked if he wanted to join any of the day's events. Mr. Siegler did not answer. He just stood in the middle of the room, looking at the floor.

"You're not going to stand there looking at the floor all day, are you?" Ben said good-naturedly.

Mr. Siegler said nothing. He just stood there silently.

Ben said, "Well, okay, I'll go now. But if you want to join an activity, just come and do it. We'll be glad to have you." Then Ben left.

It is hard to evaluate Mr. Siegler's experience of the interaction with Ben. Mr. Siegler often said or did little because he did not want to reveal what he was feeling or thinking. Only when he felt safe with someone was Mr. Siegler able to describe his fears. It typically took repeated, brief contact with a person before Mr. Siegler felt safe.

Interacting with Ben was new to Mr. Siegler. Being approached by a stranger likely heightened Mr. Siegler's fear and suspicion and contributed to his silence and inactivity.

Coping with Stress

From your own experience, the examples of Mrs. Wells, Ms. Quigley, Mr. D'Angelo, and Mr. Siegler may seem familiar. You may recognize that what people in need of care do or say often provokes a variety of reactions in caregivers and others (for example, long-term care staff members such as housekeepers, food service workers, chaplains, and pharmacists). Some of our reactions as caregivers or staff members—whether they are feelings such as frustration, fear, anger, or depression—will, if they are strong enough, cause us stress.

Our roles as caregivers, however, are not the only source of stress. At times we also feel stress related to different obligations, such as to our families and others. All of these potential sources of stress add to our overall stress level, making it difficult to cope effectively with any particular stressful situation, such as dealing with a care recipient's challenging behavior.

Justine's Experience

Justine, a licensed practical nurse (LPN) who worked at a long-term care facility, was a single mother with a 7-year-old daughter, Katie. Her own mother had recently had a stroke, and Justine visited her daily at the hospital.

Before work one morning, Justine had an argument during a telephone conversation with her ex-husband. They argued about which parent would pick up Katie after school and take her to Justine's sister's house while Justine visited her mother at the hospital. Although her ex-husband finally agreed to pick up their daughter that afternoon, the argument had taken so much time that Justine was afraid that she would be late for work.

When Justine was about to go out the door with Katie, she remembered that she needed to pay for her daughter's school lunch program. While quickly writing a check, she noticed that her checking account was overdrawn.

As Justine was leaving Katie at the school's early morning child care program, the principal greeted her. She wanted to talk to Justine about Katie having pushed another child down during recess the day before. The principal was concerned, she said, because Justine's daughter had acted similarly a number of times recently. After promising to call for an appointment to discuss all of this at another time, Justine drove to work. She was sure that she would be late.

Justine was really only 5 minutes late. She was relieved when no one seemed concerned. In fact, her supervisor gave her a warm, "Hello, Justine." A moment later, her friend, another LPN, said, "Hey, girlfriend. I'm calling the take-out place early to have some food delivered for lunchtime. Do you want me to order your usual?" The unit secretary looked up to say hello and added how nice Justine's new hairstyle looked.

With the way the day had started, Justine had been nearly ready to scream or cry when she arrived at work. She gratefully considered how the brief pleasant interactions with her supervisor, her friend, and the unit secretary were just what she needed. Although not completely over the difficulties of the morning, Justine did feel a little less tense and upset. She appreciated the slight positive shift in her mood.

Having to interact with Mr. D'Angelo without those small pleasant events might have been the last straw for Justine. Without the boost from those interactions, she might have reacted in a less-than-positive way. As it turned out, she effectively responded to Mr. D'Angelo when he said, "What are you doing? Get the hell outta here!" while turning his head to avoid the medications she was trying to give him. She gently said that she would come back a little later to see if he was ready for his medications then.

It also helped her respond to Ms. Quigley. While Justine was giving medications to Ms. Quigley's next-door neighbors, Ms. Quigley stuck her head out her door three times in 15 minutes to ask, "When is it time for my medication?" Justine answered her quietly each time, first saying that Ms. Quigley's medication would be given in the next 20 minutes, then saying the next 15 minutes, and finally saying, "Right now, Ms. Quigley. Here you go."

The effects of Justine's brief positive interactions with other staff members— simply small, pleasant events—were not major. However, they helped balance the stressful experiences of that morning. This made it more likely that Justine would effectively address difficult situations that might arise. Applying the following method of using small, pleasant events could help you manage stress in your days.

Using Pleasant Events to Manage Stress

Pleasant events are activities that you enjoy. They can be small, everyday experiences. Having someone smile at you, preparing a tasty meal, laughing, or taking a walk are examples of pleasant events. Although these events are small, having many throughout the day can be very helpful in counteracting stress.

Setting a Goal

How many pleasant activities should you have each day? Only you can decide the answer to this question. It may be good to strive for a balance between the number of pleasant activities that you experience and the more difficult tasks that you are obligated to do. A sign that you have reached this balance is that you do not feel burned out or overly stressed.

The research of psychologist Peter Lewinsohn and his colleagues suggests that the average adult has between five and ten pleasant events a day. You can use this range as a guide. If you are having fewer than five pleasant experiences a day, you may want to increase the number. If you are having as many as ten pleasant events per day, you are not likely to be overindulging. Also, you may need additional pleasant events during particularly stressful times. When your circumstances are notably stressful, it is good to plan for more than five to ten pleasant activities each day. This may foster a balance that will help protect your mental and physical health and positively affect your work and relationships with others. Keep in mind that providing care or working in a long-term care setting is likely, at least occasionally, to put you in circumstances that are more stressful than the experiences of the average person.

Increasing Your Pleasant Events

The list that follows outlines a method for increasing the number of pleasant events that you have each day.

Making Your List of Pleasant Events. Use the Top 10 Pleasant Events List (or "Top 10 List") in the appendix at the end of the book to make a list of 10 activities you enjoy doing. Make sure that you include what you can realistically do. For example, a 2-month cruise to faraway places is less realistic than going to a favorite neighborhood coffee shop, taking a walk, reading, or sitting quietly for a few minutes. See Handout 1.2 for a list of activities many people find enjoyable.

In addition to being realistic, activities should not be ones that you already do often. Your list will then include the top 10 "do-able" pleasant activities that you can do on a regular basis. Rank the items, putting the most pleasant, do-able, and infrequent activity at the top of the list. Do-able activities that you do not engage in much are likely to be those that you stand an excellent chance of adding to your day to increase your number of pleasant events.

Tracking Pleasant Events. Over the course of a week, use the Pleasant Events Tracking Form in the appendix to note which days you engaged in each top 10 activity so that you can look back and see how many of your top activities you actually engaged in each day.

Revising Your Top 10 List. After a week of tracking your Top 10 List, determine if it needs some changes. Were you unable to do a particular activity? Would a different activity be more realistic? Use the New Top 10 List of Pleasant Events form in the appendix to make a revised list. Replace anything on your original list that you were not able to do.

Tracking Your New Top 10. Over the course of the next week, use the Pleasant Events Tracking Form in the appendix again. See how many of these pleasant activities you engage in each day.

Continuing with Pleasant Events. Each week you can revise your list by following the preceding two steps. Eventually, you may find that making a list is unnecessary because you have learned to include enough pleasant events in your life. However, if you begin to feel overwhelmed, tense, or depressed, or if you begin to notice any other signs of stress, it can be helpful to once again follow this method for increasing pleasant events.

Planning Ahead. Planning ahead can help you increase your number of enjoyable activities. If an activity involves taking a trip or going out for an evening, you might have to think ahead. For example, to plan your route, buy tickets for an event, or arrange for a babysitter. If an activity cuts into time for activities that you do not enjoy, such as housecleaning or shopping, you will need to make plans for tending to these chores.

Some enjoyable activities are easier to work into a busy schedule and require less planning. On full days, it may be good to do those less complicated pleasant activities. Also, once you have planned a pleasant activity, you might face pressure from others to give up your plan. Remember that it is usually okay to say, "Sorry, but I have other plans during that time."

Summary

Chapter 1 discussed the following five major influences on the behavior of those who need close attention and care:

- *Physical functioning:* How a person's body (including the brain) functioning contributes to behavior.

- *Emotions:* How someone feels emotionally is a primary influence on the way he or she acts.

- *Thinking:* The way that an individual thinks about or understands what is happening to or around him or her affects behavior.

- *Behavior:* Some behaviors lead to other behaviors, and some behaviors seem to perpetuate themselves.

- *Interactions with other people:* The way that a person experiences interactions with other people has a significant influence on his or her behavior.

The chapter also emphasized the importance of remembering that every challenging behavior is likely to have internal and external causes.

Finally, Chapter 1 raised the idea that our stress level can affect how well we cope with difficult situations. Increasing our number of small, daily pleasant activities is an approach to stress management.

Understanding Causes of Challenging Behaviors

A *challenging behavior* is any behavior that is harmful physically or emotionally. It can be harmful to the person doing it or to someone else. Examples of challenging behaviors include a depressed person withdrawing from other people, an agitated person shouting repeatedly or hitting someone, or a confused individual wandering and getting lost.

Causes of challenging behaviors include internal and external factors that combine to trigger or reinforce a behavior.

Sample internal triggers or reinforcers	Sample external triggers or reinforcers
Emotion (e.g., despair, anxiety, fear)	Lack of meaningful activity
Medication	Unpleasant events
Illness (physical or mental)	Unpleasant actions of others
Confusion	Demands of others
Pain or discomfort	Light that is too bright or too dim
Lifelong perceptions	Too much noise
	Being misunderstood by others

Remember: Every challenging behavior is likely to have both internal and external causes.

Pleasant Events

Pleasant events are activities that you enjoy. They can range from getting a hug, to watching the sunset, to enjoying a favorite television program. Experiencing pleasant events throughout the day can help us deal with stress. The positive effects of frequent pleasant activities can help balance the negative impacts of stressful circumstances.

Examples of Events Many People Find Pleasant*

Laughing	Breathing clean air	Spending time with friends
Spending time in the country	Kissing	Sitting in the sun
Hearing that I am loved	Having a lively talk	Having a good meal
Wearing clean clothes	Being with someone I love	Amusing people
Watching people	Being with pets	Having sex
Reading	Driving	Having spare time
Smiling at people	Seeing old friends	Being relaxed
Expressing my love	Complimenting someone	Going to a party
Being seen as attractive	Viewing wild animals	Sleeping well
Being complimented	Thinking about people I like	Learning
Planning or organizing	Having a frank discussion	Speaking clearly
Doing a project my way	Seeing beautiful scenery	Doing a job well

*Source: Lewinsohn, Muñoz, Youngren, & Zeiss (1986).

If you are having as many as 10 such experiences per day, it is unlikely that you are overindulging. If you are having fewer than 5, you may be at risk of suffering the negative mental and physical effects of stress.

When life is more stressful than usual for you, it is a good idea to plan more than the average number of pleasant activities each day.

EXERCISE 1.1

Think about an incident in which someone in your care engaged in a challenging behavior. If you cannot think of an incident involving someone receiving care from you, think of one in which someone else behaved in a difficult way. Remember, a difficult behavior is a behavior that is harmful to someone in some way. It may be harmful to the person engaging in the behavior or to someone else. The harm can be either physical or emotional.

Briefly describe the incident.

Briefly describe the following:

1. What seemed to be some of the internal triggers for the challenging behavior?

2. What were some possible external triggers of the challenging behavior?

Encouraging Positive Behaviors

One of the most significant influences on the behavior of someone who needs close care and attention is external: It is *our* behavior, particularly our behavior around the person and how we behave toward him or her, that often impacts the care recipient's actions and responses. Through our actions, we can encourage those who depend on our care to behave in positive ways and, at the same time, decrease or eliminate challenging, or difficult, behaviors. The more someone is engaged in positive behaviors, the less the person will engage in challenging behaviors. In fact, the best way to reduce challenging behaviors is to encourage, trigger, or reinforce positive behaviors. The single most important source of encouragement or reinforcement for positive behavior is us, the people upon whom those in need of care must depend. This chapter looks at three ways of encouraging and reinforcing positive behaviors: engaging in active listening; allowing choices; and using praise, compliments, and acknowledgment. Chapter 2 also continues to focus on ways of coping with stress as well as describes the stress management technique of progressive muscle relaxation.

Engaging in Active Listening

The way that we communicate with those who need our care can promote positive behavior. One group of very effective communication skills is called *active listening.* When we use active listening effectively, we tune in to the thoughts and feelings of the person we are listening to. When we use these techniques, we are able to increase our empathic understanding of those who depend on our care. Effective use of active listening can communicate that we hear what the person needs us to hear. It also lets the person know that we can tolerate and accept who he or she is and what he or she feels or experiences.

Generally, the more people experience being listened to in this way (frequently described as *feeling emotionally supported*), the more positive their behaviors become. This type of emotional social support is associated with mental and physical health as well as overall quality of life. It appears to be a basic human need, much like an essential nutrient, with powerful effects on physical, psychological, and behavioral functioning. There can be striking ill effects of "undernourishment" when this support is in short supply. Behavioral, psychological, and physical problems are likely to worsen, especially in those who are most vulnerable due to predisposition, stress, or illness. These are the people who most need the "nutrient" of accurate emotional attunement.

Unfortunately, challenging behaviors frequently discourage others from providing close, accepting support. Often, we are more likely to respond by withdrawing from or avoiding a person who engages in challenging behaviors. However, this can result in a negative cycle of worsening behavior and further withdrawal or avoidance.

By using active listening, we can help care recipients meet their needs for basic human emotional support and encourage positive behaviors. When we use active listening, we stop what we are doing and show that we are paying attention to the person. We make eye contact, to the degree the person is able to tolerate. We use body language to show that we are listening: we nod, sit, crouch, or bend down to be at eye level with people who are in wheelchairs, geriatric chairs, or beds. We show that we are listening by saying "Hmm," "Uh-huh," and "Oh." We also summarize and restate what the person says or feels.

Offering advice, making suggestions, correcting the speaker's misperceptions, or telling the speaker what to do are not parts of active listening. Although these responses may be important at times, they should come only after we use active listening, if at all. Typically, it is best to spend more time actively listening than giving advice, making suggestions, correcting misperceptions, or telling others what to do. Frequently, our being truly present and accepting is of greater importance than attempting to solve others' problems or making their troubling emotions go away. See Handout 2.1 for a summary of active listening and the following case studies for illustrations of these skills.

Mrs. Ortiz

At age 83, Mrs. Ortiz was very forgetful. Whenever she left her room at the long-term care facility, she could not remember how to get back. Sometimes she was found sitting in someone else's room. She frequently misplaced her possessions and lost money. Still, Mrs. Ortiz liked to have a few dollars handy. She agreed with her treatment team and family's decision to give her a small amount of cash each week.

One day, Mrs. Ortiz used all of her cash to buy some toiletries. Later, when Phil, a staff social worker, asked Mrs. Ortiz how she was doing, she looked up from her wheelchair and said, "They keep taking my money."

"You've lost some money," Phil responded.

"I didn't lose anything. These people here took it. They take *everything*!" Mrs. Ortiz said as she shook her fist in the air.

"I don't think anyone took your money, Mrs. Ortiz. You spent it this morning," Phil said.

"You don't think! You don't think!" Mrs. Ortiz said, raising her voice and shaking both fists at Phil. There were tears in her eyes.

"It can be pretty hard when no one seems to believe you," Phil stated, voicing what he thought was Mrs. Ortiz's point of view.

"That's right," said Mrs. Ortiz, putting down her fists. "They take all of your things and then cover up for each other," she continued.

"You're having all of your things taken and nobody is admitting it," Phil said, restating what Mrs. Ortiz just said.

"Oh, dear, I miss my things," Mrs. Ortiz said, crying quietly. "I used to have such nice things."

Phil crouched down to eye level with Mrs. Ortiz and held her hand. "It's very sad, not having your things," he said. With this reply, Phil named the feeling that he believed Mrs. Ortiz was experiencing and restated her apparent explanation for her behavior.

"You're such a nice man," Mrs. Ortiz said, patting Phil's hand.

"Thank you. I like talking with you, too," Phil said.

After a moment, Phil said he had to go but that he would stop by again later in the day.

"Oh, I'd like that, dear," Mrs. Ortiz responded. "But what about my money?"

"Maybe we can talk more about that when I see you again," Phil answered.

"Okay," said Mrs. Ortiz.

This situation started out a bit rocky. When Phil tried to convince Mrs. Ortiz that her money had not been stolen, she became agitated. Phil de-escalated the situation by using the active listening techniques of stating what he thought Mrs. Ortiz believed and restating what he heard her say. He used body language to show that he was listening by crouching down to eye level and holding Mrs. Ortiz's hand. Phil also used the active listening technique of naming the feeling he thought Mrs. Ortiz was having when he said, "It's very sad. . . ."

Phil effectively encouraged Mrs. Ortiz's positive behavior of talking with him about what was happening from her point of view. Although what Mrs. Ortiz was saying about others seemed untrue, talking about her beliefs, point of view, and feelings were positive behaviors. Phil's use of active listening also encouraged Mrs. Ortiz to speak less loudly and to cease using threatening hand gestures.

It is not unusual for someone in circumstances like Mrs. Ortiz's to become agitated when another person denies what he or she believes is real. When a resident is very confused and agitated, trying to convince him or her of our version of the truth—that is, trying to orient the person to reality—will not usually reassure the person. More likely, it will increase that individual's confusion. Often, this triggers the person to fight against the confusion by insisting on the rightness of his or her point of view. It can also lead to increasing agitation. If a care recipient is more prone to feeling victimized than confused, he or she may react to attempts to correct misperceptions as further victimization. The person may feel that his or her reality is being denied, and his or her ability to think clearly is being attacked. Frequently, the more attacked someone feels, the more inclined he or she is to counterattack in defense. Phil avoided all of these possible problems by using active listening.

When Phil was first learning to use active listening, it was uncomfortable for him. To him, reflecting back, restating, echoing, or mirroring what a resident said often seemed like lying. When Phil was learning active listening techniques, he would not have been able to say, "You're having all of your things taken and nobody is admitting it" in response to Mrs. Ortiz's statement that "They take all of your things and then cover up for each other." Back then, Phil would have thought this response meant he agreed with the statement. It was not until he started trying the techniques of restating and rephrasing that he understood their value. Phil eventually recognized that using these listening techniques did not necessarily mean that he agreed with the words he used when he restated or rephrased what he heard.

As he used active listening over time, Phil also realized that truths typically underlie the specific words used in an interaction such as the one with Mrs. Ortiz. For example, Mrs. Ortiz *did* feel sad. Although staff members were not taking her things, something was being taken from her—her physical and cognitive functioning. All of this was unmistakably true, unmistakably real. This was the underlying truth that Phil would not have been able to hear or understand if he had tried to defend himself and others from Mrs. Ortiz's accusations instead of engaging in active listening. If Phil had argued with Mrs. Ortiz about the details of her comments, he would not have heard deeper meaning in what she was saying. If Phil had avoided Mrs. Ortiz to escape being accused or treated like an accomplice, he would not have heard her. If Phil had reacted in these ways instead of actively listening to Mrs. Ortiz, he would have missed an opportunity to provide care for her mental health.

Behind the specific words used by a distressed or angry resident are feelings and thoughts that are very real. Sometimes illness, personality, stress, or simply lack of practice can make it difficult for people to bear these strong feelings and accurately put them into words. Those in need of care use words to express feelings that might not be literally true, but the same cannot be said for all of us. For example, when we say something like, "My heart is breaking," we do not mean that our heart is physically being broken. However, we *are* speaking of an experience that to us is very real and difficult to describe in any other words.

Active listening allows us to hear the deeper meaning of what others say. With practice, active listening can help us better understand what another person is feeling by putting us in touch with those feelings. Such empathy or emotional understanding on our part can encourage positive behaviors from those who depend on our care. This is what happened between Phil and Mrs. Ortiz.

When Phil went back to visit Mrs. Ortiz later that day, she again spoke of her money being stolen and how she wanted it replaced. Phil did not make plans with her to replace the money she said was stolen. He also did not try to convince her that it had not been stolen. He did not remind her that she had memory problems and that a plan was already in place to ensure she had spending money every week. All of these approaches had been unsuccessful with Mrs. Ortiz in the past. They usually resulted in her shouting accusations and shaking her fists. Once, Mrs. Ortiz even hit a staff member who was persistent in using such an approach to "reality orientation."

Phil made active listening his primary way of interacting with Mrs. Ortiz. As other staff members followed Phil's example, Mrs. Ortiz's episodes of angry, agitated behavior decreased and became rare. Generally, after less than a minute of active listening, Mrs. Ortiz ceased speaking of things being stolen from her. Instead, she would begin reminiscing and talking about how difficult it had been to manage her household finances during hard times as a young mother. She would then speak of her children and her husband and say how much she loved them. Mrs. Ortiz would often mention how much the person using active listening reminded her of her husband or one of her children.

Ms. Chen

Ms. Chen was 77 years old. She had lived in psychiatric units much of her life before coming to the long-term care community. Other than her mental illness, she seemed to have no disabilities. However, she was incontinent of bowel and bladder and preferred to use a wheelchair even though she could walk. Ms. Chen's psychiatric condition was usually stable, but her ability to think clearly and to interact with others had not been good for many years.

Reverend White, who frequently visited the long-term care community, was passing Ms. Chen in the hallway. He was on his way to a meeting.

"Run me over! Run me over! Run me over, why don't you!" shouted Ms. Chen, staring directly at the reverend.

"Run you over?" Reverend White asked as he stopped and looked at Ms. Chen.

"You people are all alike—always busy, busy. Never any time to make sure you're not running people over," Ms. Chen continued.

"You want me to have time for you," Reverend White said, restating what he thought Ms. Chen was saying.

"Nobody has any respect for rank and privilege around here. I'm not only wealthy; my mother is royalty. My father is, too. But we don't like to talk about that."

"You aren't being treated the way you should be," Reverend White said, summarizing Ms. Chen's statements.

"That's what I'm saying," Ms. Chen replied quietly. Then she said, "I think it's lunchtime," as she began pushing herself toward the dining room, leaving Reverend White.

Reverend White used a few active listening techniques in his interaction with Ms. Chen. He showed that he was paying attention to Ms. Chen by stopping and looking at her. When he restated and summarized what he thought she was saying, he showed that he was paying attention. In turn, Ms. Chen's shouting stopped. His continued attention to Ms. Chen during the interaction appeared to reinforce her more positive, quiet behavior. Ms. Chen had frequently shouted at people, but once staff members started regularly using active listening before she shouted, her episodes of shouting were rare.

The interaction between Reverend White and Ms. Chen was brief. There was not enough time for Reverend White to do much, as he was expected at a meeting. Yet, the discussion ended because Ms. Chen seemed to want it to. Reverend White showed that he was paying attention to that wish by not insisting that Ms. Chen say more. He did not try to find out more about Ms. Chen or to make small talk. He could do that another time. Regardless, he probably found out more about Ms. Chen by paying attention to what she did and when she did it rather than by asking her directly.

Brief, frequent interactions are often all that people with severe mental illness are able to tolerate without becoming anxious, more confused, or agitated. However, over time, gradual improvement is possible. Active listening can encourage positive behaviors, such as longer interactions with others and conversations containing fewer signs of confused thinking or delusions.

Ms. Zabransky

Ms. Zabransky, age 49, had multiple sclerosis. She needed help with all of her routine activities of daily living.

Jill, a nursing assistant, responded to Ms. Zabransky's call bell.

"It's about time you got here! I could be lying on the floor dead before you decided to come!" Ms. Zabransky yelled.

Jill said, "You feel like you've been waiting a very long time."

"I don't FEEL like anything. I WAS waiting a long f——ing time," Ms. Zabransky growled.

"You're pretty angry," Jill responded.

"Damn right, I'm angry. Wouldn't you be if you had to rely on people you can't rely on?" Ms. Zabransky went on.

"It's not easy to depend on other people when they might not be there when you need them," said Jill.

"That's right," Ms. Zabransky said, no longer yelling or growling.

"What can I do for you now?" Jill asked.

"Change the TV channel to 7," Ms. Zabransky said flatly.

Jill changed the channel and said, "It's hard when you need someone else to do something like change the TV channel."

After a pause, Ms. Zabransky said, "Yeah."

"Do you need anything else before I go?" Jill asked.

"I used to be able to do 10 different things for 10 different people at the same time," Ms. Zabransky muttered. "Now I can't even change the damned TV channel."

"Being able to do things for yourself and others is important to you. You regret that you can't do that the way you used to," Jill added.

"Yeah . . . never mind," Ms. Zabransky responded.

"Can I sit with you for a minute before I go?" Jill asked.

"No, I'm all right," answered Ms. Zabransky.

"Okay. See you later," Jill said as she left.

It can be difficult to use active listening skills. Sometimes people we provide close care and attention to communicate in hostile ways that can be hard on caregivers. It is good to keep in mind that a care recipient who is behaving in a hostile way is not, at that moment, able to contain angry feelings. Those feelings may come out in behaviors such as hurling insults, shouting, or using strong language. In such cases, it is important to make every effort to stay calm and contain our own angry or defensive reactions. It is natural to feel anger, confusion, or even fear while being verbally attacked. However, showing hostility in response to displays of hostility is likely to create a negative cycle of increasingly difficult behavior. Acting defensively, by insisting that we did nothing wrong, while the person in our care is insisting that we did usually creates a negative cycle, too.

If we react out of anger over being attacked, we may also counterattack. We may feel justified in telling off someone who behaves like Ms. Zabransky by saying things like, "Just who do you think you are?! You can't talk to me that way! All you wanted was the channel changed! If you talk to me that way again, you'll *really* wait when you push that call button!"

If a person does "behave" in response to such a reaction from us, it is likely out of intimidation. Intimidation is not a good way of promoting optimally positive behavior and good mental or physical health. Intimidation or negative consequences, such as being ignored, being avoided, or having privileges withheld, can undermine the kind of emotionally supportive interactions and relationships that encourage positive behavior, mental health, and physical health.

Trying to explain to an upset or confused individual why we are not at fault for his or her difficulties often leads to further confusion, upset feelings, or agitated behavior. In such situations, active listening is typically more helpful than saying, "You weren't waiting that long," "I have other people I need to help, too," or "I came as soon as you pushed the call button."

Jill did not react to Ms. Zabransky by counterattacking or being defensive. She did feel angry, confused, hurt, and frightened during the interaction with Ms. Zabransky. However, she was able to contain these feelings and not act on them. Later, she thought it was interesting that Ms. Zabransky was probably unable to contain similar feelings. Jill guessed that Ms. Zabransky's worsening physical condition, as well as she being alone most of the time and having lost so many of her abilities, left her feeling angry, confused, hurt, and frightened. Jill suspected that being overwhelmed by such feelings and being unable to contain them prompted the feelings to come out in Ms. Zabransky's behavior. Luckily, Jill was able to contain herself and act as a container for what Ms. Zabransky could not contain. Drawing on Jill's strength, Ms. Zabransky regained her fragile composure.

By sharing feelings, even those behind hostile behavior, the people in our care are often less burdened by them. When residents are less burdened by such feelings, their behavior typically improves.

Mr. Callahan

At age 79, long-term care community resident Mr. Callahan was recovering from a stroke. His recovery had progressed well, but after approximately 2 months, he still had not regained full use of his left hand and arm.

Mr. Callahan frequently complained that he was not treated well. He often insulted people—sometimes other residents but mostly staff. His family members said that he had always been this way. They said that he looked for faults in others and was never satisfied. They also reported that he made many demands but was rarely happy when his requests were fulfilled. Although Mr. Callahan frequently argued with and insulted people, his family noted that he hated to be alone. Mr. Callahan's behavior led many people to see him as mean, nasty, and even hateful. His behavior often elicited very strong reactions from other people.

One night, Don, a nursing assistant, was checking on Mr. Callahan's roommate, who could barely move because of a degenerative neurological condition. Mr. Callahan was asleep until Don started changing the roommate's soiled pajamas.

"You no good son of a b———! What the f—— are you doing now, you G— d—— idiot?!" Mr. Callahan yelled.

"I know I woke you up, Mr. Callahan. I tried to be as quiet as I could," Don explained.

"You're useless! You stupid sh—!" Mr. Callahan went on.

Because of all the noise, Carmela, another nursing assistant, came in to help out. She quietly continued assisting Mr. Callahan's roommate as Don addressed Mr. Callahan.

Don stated what he thought Mr. Callahan was thinking: "It doesn't do you any good for me to come in the middle of the night and wake you up while I help your roommate."

"That jerk. All the nurses take care of him. What about me?! Nobody gives a G— d—— about what I need!" Mr. Callahan continued loudly, although no longer yelling.

"It doesn't seem like anyone cares about your needs," Don said, restating Mr. Callahan's apparent reason for his feelings. Don stopped what he was doing and stood by Mr. Callahan's bedside, making eye contact with him.

"This whole place stinks," Mr. Callahan said in a much quieter tone while Carmela, who had finished her task, left.

"I'm sorry I woke you up," Don said as he straightened the cover of Mr. Callahan's bed. Then Don left the room and Mr. Callahan remained quiet for the rest of the night.

That was great teamwork by Don and Carmela. Carmela's help gave Don the time he needed to respond to Mr. Callahan effectively, in a way that reduced the intensity of Mr. Callahan's difficult behavior. Don handled a challenging situation with great skill. He used the active listening technique of restating what appeared to be Mr. Callahan's underlying reasons for his strong feelings. This helped to limit Mr. Callahan's abusive behavior. Mr. Callahan's behavior became less intense, then ceased when Don left the room.

When Don restated what Mr. Callahan seemed to be saying, he showed that he was listening to Mr. Callahan. When Don stopped what he was doing and went to Mr. Callahan's bedside, he also nonverbally signaled that he was listening. Even leaving the room as quickly as possible was a nonverbal way of Don showing that he was listening. It demonstrated that Don understood Mr. Callahan's statement about how having his sleep disrupted was another example of his needs not being considered.

By the time Don left the room, Mr. Callahan's behavior had improved. If Don had ignored Mr. Callahan, insisted that Mr. Callahan not speak to him that way, or demanded that he stop disturbing everyone else, Mr. Callahan's challenging behavior probably would have worsened. When such approaches were tried in the past, Mr. Callahan's difficult behavior escalated to the point that he was described as totally out of control. In one such situation, he threw a pitcher of water at a staff member while screaming, "I'll kill you!"

Expecting Mr. Callahan to speak in a pleasant, respectful way would have been unrealistic. Don was satisfied with the more realistic goals of helping Mr. Callahan to speak less loudly and decreasing the number of unpleasant comments he made. By using active listening techniques, Don encouraged Mr. Callahan to behave in a less difficult way. In this case, the positive behavior fostered was simply the change from very difficult behavior to less difficult behavior. The situation ended with Mr. Callahan spending the remainder of the night resting quietly.

The more that staff members used active listening in response to Mr. Callahan's complaints, insults, and threats, the less loud, insulting, and threatening his behavior became. Although Mr. Callahan still displayed some challenging behaviors, they happened less often and were usually not extreme. Also, difficult episodes with Mr. Callahan had initially happened several times a day. Eventually, they rarely happened more than twice per week.

Mrs. Lowenthal

Mrs. Lowenthal was 100 years old. She had lived in the long-term care community for a year. Mrs. Lowenthal was almost completely blind and not strong enough to stand and walk on her own. Although her hearing was greatly impaired, hearing aids helped somewhat. Mrs. Lowenthal was an intelligent woman and had no life-threatening illnesses. However, she was taking a number of medications for ongoing health problems.

Mrs. Lowenthal had seemed depressed for some time, but refused to try medication for depression. She also said she did not see the point of talking to a psychologist or any other mental health professional.

Mrs. Lowenthal sometimes said she was tired of living and wished she would die. However, when asked if she would ever take her own life, she clearly stated that she would never do such a thing.

One day Teresa, an LPN, was giving Mrs. Lowenthal her medications. As Mrs. Lowenthal swallowed them, she said, "I'll take them, but I don't see the point."

Teresa restated what Mrs. Lowenthal said: "You don't see the point of taking your medicine."

"That's right. I don't see the point. I think this is too much fuss for someone who's been around long enough," said Mrs. Lowenthal.

"You've had a long life and you think it's been long enough," Teresa summarized.

"Well," continued Mrs. Lowenthal, "I'm blind. I'm losing my hearing. I can't even go to the toilet without help."

"You've lost so much," Teresa responded.

"That's right. I'm no use to anyone. If I got the wrong medicine and I never woke up, I would be better off," Mrs. Lowenthal said.

"You feel pretty worthless and ready to die. You're very unhappy," Teresa said. After a brief pause, she asked, "How do you feel about our talking like this?"

"I think about these things all the time. And nobody wants to hear it," Mrs. Lowenthal said as she sighed very deeply. "They ask how I'm doing, but they don't want to hear it. Not really. It's too much for them. They tell me to think about the positive things or to remember the good times. Sometimes they even say, 'Oh, Mrs. Lowenthal, I can't stand to hear what is happening to you.' Nobody knows what's happening to me. Nobody wants to know because it's too overwhelming for them. They even avoid coming to see me because it's hard for them to see what being old is like. I'm a burden . . . but you'd better go, dear. I know you have other things to do."

Teresa restated what she thought Mrs. Lowenthal meant: "You think you're burdening me."

"Well, yes. But I do know you have your work to do."

Teresa took Mrs. Lowenthal's hand and gave it a gentle squeeze. "I do need to go now, but I'll see you when I come back a little later," she said.

"Thank you, dear," responded Mrs. Lowenthal.

Teresa did an excellent job. She briefly stopped delivering medications. She restated and summarized what she thought Mrs. Lowenthal was saying. She also asked the open-ended question, "How do you feel about our talking like this?" Unlike yes-or-no or either-or questions, the occasional open-ended question can help when we are using active listening. It shows the person that we are listening and that we are available and interested in hearing what he or she has to say.

Teresa's question helped her determine how their conversation was affecting Mrs. Lowenthal. Teresa had suspected that talking this way was only making Mrs. Lowenthal feel worse. However, Teresa found out that it was actually helping Mrs. Lowenthal, who had believed that no one—including Teresa—wanted to listen to her.

Teresa realized that both she and Mrs. Lowenthal had been afraid that the other was feeling overwhelmed. Teresa acknowledged to herself that it *was* hard for her to witness the end-of-life experience that was nearly overtaking Mrs. Lowenthal. It upset Teresa to think of how desolate it must feel to be in such circumstances: failing eyesight, diminishing hearing, continually decreasing mobility, being alone most of the time, and waiting for death. It was potentially overwhelming for Teresa to be in touch with what was happening to Mrs. Lowenthal.

Empathically understanding someone else requires feeling some of what the person feels. Mrs. Lowenthal's experience was that no one wanted to be close enough to her to understand her in this way. When others told her to think positively and remember good times or said they could not stand to hear what was happening to her, she believed that they were trying to avoid being overwhelmed by her experience. It left her feeling very alone.

However, even though she wanted support from others, Mrs. Lowenthal prompted people to leave her alone, just as she tried to get Teresa to go on with her work. In future interactions, by using active listening and accepting the feelings that she encountered, Teresa encouraged Mrs. Lowenthal to talk more about herself, her feelings, her experience, her life, and her death. When she talked this way, Mrs. Lowenthal felt less alone and depressed. Shortly before she died, Mrs. Lowenthal thanked Teresa and said that because of her, she would not feel quite so alone when she died.

Teresa's use of active listening encouraged Mrs. Lowenthal's positive behavior of talking about her thoughts and feelings. It also increased Mrs. Lowenthal's interactions with others. These positive behaviors replaced her challenging behavior of isolating herself because of depression.

Mr. Deuval

Mr. Deuval, age 73 and a long-term care community resident, had his left leg amputated below the knee because of diabetes. Approximately 6 months later, he was diagnosed with a fast-growing cancer that had already spread throughout much of his body. He was not expected to live much longer.

Mr. Deuval seemed very depressed. His treatment involved taking antidepressant medication and having weekly visits from the unit social worker. The recreation therapist checked in with Mr. Deuval occasionally, hoping that he would become more actively involved in therapeutic recreation. The chaplain also visited periodically.

One day when Mr. Deuval was alone in his room, Alma, a nursing assistant, came in to make his bed. "How are you this morning, Mr. Deuval?" she asked cheerfully. Mr. Deuval sat in his wheelchair without replying. Alma quietly finished making the bed, then said, "It's a beautiful day." Mr. Deuval still said nothing. Alma commented, "I guess you don't feel much like talking now—or maybe it is too hard for you to talk right now." When she was done straightening up the room, she said, "You seem to be feeling very down. Could I sit with you for just a minute before I leave?" Mr. Deuval did not answer. He looked at her and then looked away. "I'll sit for just a minute," Alma said, "If you want me to go, just say so." She sat in a chair and looked out the window for a minute. Then she got up and said good-bye. As she was walking out the door, Mr. Deuval said, "Thank you."

"You're very welcome, Mr. Deuval," Alma responded.

In this example, Alma "listened" to Mr. Deuval's nonverbal communication. She accepted what he was feeling when she did not try to convince him to talk or to "snap out of it." She made it clear that she was listening to Mr. Deuval when she took a minute to just sit with him. Alma also showed that she was paying attention when she stated what she thought his nonverbal communication might mean: "I guess you don't feel much like talking now—or maybe it is too hard for you to talk right now." Naming Mr. Deuval's feeling ("you seem to be feeling very down") was another way that Alma showed she was paying attention to Mr. Deuval.

Alma did not make suggestions, give advice, reassure, or offer a different way of looking at things. This was a good approach. After all, Mr. Deuval's silence made it hard to know what to suggest, advise, reassure, or offer.

Overall, Alma did a very good job. She respected and tolerated Mr. Deuval's feelings. In doing this, she seemed to help him feel less isolated and decrease his withdrawn behavior, even if only slightly.

Active listening calls for accepting what a person is expressing. When people are listened to in this way, they typically feel accepted and respected, as though they matter or have worth. What they think and feel, what they experience as who they are, is seen, accepted, or tolerated as we listen empathically. Being listened to in this way encourages positive behavior. It also may soothe confused, angry, agitated, or depressed people. Our ability to engage in interactions with such individuals depends largely on our ability to tolerate our own feelings as we accept their emotions. That means working to tolerate the feelings, instead of avoiding them, denying them, acting them out, or being overwhelmed by them. For example, we may feel anger in response to someone who angrily shouts, criticizes, blames, or threatens. Yet, if we are too uncomfortable to acknowledge our own anger to ourselves, are too frightened by the strength of our reaction, or respond in a hostile counterattack, we will not react with empathy. In turn, we might lose an opportunity to affect positively the person in our care or decrease difficult behavior.

We can feel frightened, overwhelmed, stressed, helpless, hopeless, useless, and worthless in our work with those who need care because of their challenging behaviors, their illnesses, the circumstances of their lives, or the circumstances of their deaths. It can be difficult to contain these feelings and remain tolerant and accepting of people in our care, who frequently have similar emotions. Yet, how well we cope with these feelings influences how effectively we provide the kind of interactions where those who depend on our care feel listened to and respected in ways that promote positive behavior. Try completing Exercise 2.1 to add to your personal understanding of the ideas presented in the chapter.

Allowing Choices

Much of what someone who needs close attention and care experiences can make it difficult for him or her to feel like a capable, worthwhile individual. By the time a person needs a significant amount of care and assistance, he or she has already probably lost much, such as a home and important relationships with his or her spouse, children, friends, co-workers, and colleagues. Becoming increasingly dependent on others as one's physical and cognitive abilities decline can cause a horrifying loss of self, of who one is or is supposed to be.

Supporting and acknowledging a person's individuality or autonomy, even as both decline, can help the person cope with the sometimes overwhelming despair and fear about this sense of disintegration. As we support the person's sense of being someone of worth, we encourage positive behaviors in place of the challenging behaviors prompted by the fear, anger, and despair the person might feel because of what is happening at this stage of his or her life.

One technique for supporting a sense of worth and autonomy is allowing the individual to make choices. When we allow a person to routinely make choices, we show that we recognize the importance of his or her having a say in what is happening. Encouraging and supporting as much decision making as possible is also a way of reinforcing independent functioning and fostering cooperation with care that is necessary for optimal health. People tend to be more independently involved in and cooperative during activities and interactions in which they have some say. It is important that we support everyday decision making to the degree that an individual is interested and capable, as long as doing so does not place the person in need of care or others at immediate risk of harm.

Framing Choices

Making a choice is an independent act that can become increasingly important when illness or other circumstances make other independent acts impossible, such as routine activities of daily living. We can often encourage a resident to make choices by using open-ended questions instead of either-or or yes-or-no questions. Open-ended questions are good when we are assisting with activities of daily living, such as dressing, bathing, or eating. For example, "What time would you like to go to bed tonight?" is an open-ended question. Such questions are most helpful with those who are interested in and capable of making these decisions. If the person refuses to make a decision when given this kind of choice, consider using active listening before asking the question again.

Open-ended questions can be helpful in a variety of situations. They can support and encourage a sense of independence in those who are facing numerous treatment options for health or rehabilitation issues. They can be helpful with care recipients who are cooperative and whose thinking has not been significantly impaired by illness. Open-ended questions can also be used during therapeutic recreation and physical therapy sessions to determine which activities or exercises the care recipient prefers.

Limited-choice questions can also be used to encourage active involvement in decision making. These are yes-or-no questions ("Would you like to get out of bed now?) or either-or questions ("Would you like to get out of bed now or when I come back in 20 minutes?"). These questions, like open-ended questions, can be used with people who are interested in and able to make decisions. However, for most residents who are able and willing to make decisions and who cooperate with needed care, it is usually better to use open-ended questions more than limited-choice questions.

Limited-choice questions can be particularly helpful for those who are prone to bad moods or who are easily confused. These care recipients may not be interested in or capable of making decisions or cooperating. Yes-or-no questions often are not as helpful as either-or questions. For example, we may ask someone a yes-or-no question such as "Would you like to take a shower?" Often enough in this type of situation, a person needing to feel a sense of power or control will respond, "No." If the choices we offer are simply yes or no, no may often be selected, even though it may not be the most healthful, helpful, or considerate choice. By offering limited choices by using either-or questions we let the person know what our hope, goal, or expectation is (for example, that we will help him or her out of bed) in a way that may help reduce confusion and confrontation. However, it also allows a choice within limits, which can encourage the cooperation of someone who is inclined to resist care or is easily confused by too many options.

Whether we use open-ended questions or limited-choice questions, it is important to ask only one question at a time and wait for an answer before asking another question. This can show that we are interested and want to understand the individual's wishes.

When working with a new care recipient or one whose ability to make decisions or cooperate has improved (by, for example, effectively addressing medical conditions [such as delirium], improving psychotic symptoms, decreasing agitation, or reducing overwhelming stress), it is best to start with open-ended questions and then gauge the person's reaction. These questions could be posed during routine activities of daily living, recreational activities, or physical therapy. If the person resists or shows signs of confusion or agitation, try limited-choice questions instead.

If using the limited-choice questions does not reduce the confusion or agitation or does not engage the person's cooperation, take a break from asking questions. This could be a good time to try active listening. Once the agitation or confusion seems sufficiently reduced, try another limited-choice question. However, if the agitated or confused behavior does not decrease as you use active listening and offer choices, leave the person alone until the behavior stops (as long as doing so would not pose immediate risk to either the individual or anyone else). When immediate care is necessary, ask a co-worker or another caregiver to take over—especially one who works well in difficult situations.

Once the individual has calmed down, you can try another technique if using both types of questions does not work. This technique involves giving simple step-by-step explanations of what you are doing or what you need the person to do. For example, while holding the individual's shirt you might say, "I'll help you put on your shirt. Here we go." Then, while holding the person's wrist and guiding his or her arm, you might say, "Now, put this arm through this sleeve." When using this technique, it is important to praise effort and participation to reassure and encourage the person. Handout 2.2 summarizes how to use opportunities for allowing choices to encourage positive behavior. Exercise 2.2 is provided to help emphasize the ideas covered in this section.

Using Praise, Compliments, and Acknowledgment

Praise, compliments, and acknowledgement can be effective social reinforcers of behavior. When we praise a care recipient's actions, we encourage positive behavior by acknowledging that person's individual ability, effort, or contribution; we provide positive attention. When people regularly receive praise, they tend to feel valued and appreciated for who they are. They also frequently have warm and affectionate feelings for those who hold them in positive regard.

It is important to regularly praise and acknowledge those in our care for their positive behaviors and efforts, even for tasks that they are "just supposed to do." The case studies that follow illustrate the use of praise, compliments, and acknowledgements.

Mr. Weldon

During a particularly hectic time for the long-term care staff, Mr. Weldon, a resident, sat quietly waiting for help calling his daughter. When a staff member was able to help Mr. Weldon, she said, "Mr. Weldon, it was good of you to sit quietly while we were all so busy. It was such a calming influence. Thank you for waiting." This acknowledgment was especially important because Mr. Weldon frequently had difficulty being patient.

Mrs. Hamadi

Praising effort, and not just successful task completion, can encourage the positive behavior of continued effort.

For several days, Mrs. Hamadi had been refusing to do any of the range-of-motion exercises that her physical therapist, Jenna, recommended for rehabilitation after a stroke. When Mrs. Hamadi finally let Jenna bend and stretch her paralyzed arm, Jenna said, "Good work, Mrs. Hamadi. Good work with your exercises today." Mrs. Hamadi still refused to allow Jenna to work her affected leg. Jenna said, "Why don't we just give it a little try," as she reached for Mrs. Hamadi's leg. Mrs. Hamadi screamed until Jenna stepped back. Jenna said, "I guess you want me to listen to you when you say no the first time. I'm sorry for having gone too far. Well, you did some good work today on your arm. I'm glad we were able to work on that together."

Jenna used praise well. She did not fixate on what Mrs. Hamadi did not do or mention the screaming. Instead, Jenna praised Mrs. Hamadi's positive behavior. Jenna also used active listening by restating what she thought Mrs. Hamadi was trying to express when she screamed. Over the next few weeks, Mrs. Hamadi tolerated more bending and stretching of her arm and even began doing it on her own. Jenna then asked Mrs. Hamadi which of the recommended leg exercises she wanted to do. Mrs. Hamadi requested the one in which Jenna would lift Mrs. Hamadi's extended leg slightly as she lay on the exercise table. Jenna praised Mrs. Hamadi's positive behavior of selecting an exercise by saying, "Good choice," and then asked, "Would you like to start with that exercise or do it at the end of our session?" Mrs. Hamadi said that she would prefer to do it at the end of the session. "Great," Jenna replied, positively affirming Mrs. Hamadi's choice. Mrs. Hamadi did the exercise at the end of the session, and Jenna acknowledged this participation with a smile, a hug, and the remark, "Great work on that leg."

Mrs. Swensen

Mrs. Swensen, who was very frail and weak, asked her nursing assistant, Kara, for help getting into bed. Kara was on her way to help the resident in the next room, so she told Mrs. Swensen that she would help her in approximately 15 minutes. The wait turned out to be only 10 minutes. Although Mrs. Swensen complained that she had been kept waiting, Kara complimented Mrs. Swensen on her helpful behavior of waiting: "It's annoying to be kept waiting. Even though it is annoying, you did it, and it was a help to me that you were able to wait. Thank you." Kara also used active listening by naming Mrs. Swensen's apparent feeling (annoyance), and restating why she thought Mrs. Swensen was annoyed (she had to wait).

Using praise in combination with other techniques, such as active listening, encourages positive behavior. It can also help a person in need of care value his or her relationship with you. A valued relationship, in turn, can promote a wide range of positive behaviors. For instance, after Kara thanked Mrs. Swensen for waiting, Mrs. Swensen responded, "Oh, that's okay." Kara's skillful, empathic interaction with Mrs. Swensen continued as Kara smiled and offered Mrs. Swensen a choice about which nightgown to wear to bed.

In addition to praise, simple expressions of acknowledgment, such as regularly saying "Hello," "Good-bye," and "Thank you," can promote positive behaviors and a sense of personal worth in the people we care for. Acknowledgment can be conveyed by nonverbal means as well, such as smiling, nodding in affirmation, winking, or giving a thumbs-up sign. Giving a hug or patting a care recipient on the back, shoulder, or arm can also be warm expressions of acknowledgment. Most people who need close care and attention are likely to welcome and benefit from physical contact of this type. However, be sure to respect the wishes of those who are uncomfortable with this kind of touching. Handout 2.3 offers an overview on using praise, compliments, and acknowledgment. Exercise 2.3 presents personal applications for this section's content.

Things to Avoid When Trying to Encourage Positive Behavior

This chapter has presented ways to encourage positive behavior. Some examples have touched on what to avoid when dealing with challenging behaviors. When trying to support positive behavior, it is best to avoid showing annoyance, frustration, or anger toward someone who is behaving in a difficult way. It is also important to avoid power struggles with a person when responding to a challenging behavior. Furthermore, it is typically very unhelpful to nag, argue, or repeatedly demand that a person in need of care do something (or stop doing something). Other typically unhelpful reactions to the challenging behaviors of those we provide care to are when we threaten, tease, or laugh at the person by making him or her the butt of jokes, using sarcasm, or scolding. It is also unhelpful to give the resident "a dose of one's own medicine" by, for example, threatening an individual who makes threats, shouting at one who shouts, or insulting one who has insulted you. See Handout 2.4 for additional examples of approaches to avoid. These actions are not only likely to be ineffective, but also often trigger and reinforce challenging behaviors. Instead, it is best to support positive behavior by using techniques such as active listening, providing choices, and using praise, compliments, and acknowledgment.

Using Relaxation Techniques

As mentioned in Chapter 1, managing our own overall stress level can help us to more effectively address the challenging behaviors of care recipients. If we are not overstressed when we are confronted with a difficult situation, we are more likely to control our own emotions and respond in an empathic way.

A good way to reduce stress is to spend some time each day relaxing, clearing our minds of stressful thoughts, and releasing tension from our bodies. Setting aside 10–20 minutes per day to practice the following relaxation techniques may significantly reduce your stress level. With regular practice, many people find these methods easy, effective, and enjoyable.

First, choose a comfortable place where you will not be disturbed for 10–20 minutes. It is good to pick a regular time and place for practicing relaxation exercises, particularly when you are first learning them.

Get into a comfortable position. Sitting or lying down is fine, but you may risk falling asleep if you choose to lie down. Sleeping can sometimes help reduce stress, but the goal of these techniques is to trigger and maintain your body's ability to relax while you are awake. Staying awake while deeply relaxed takes practice—practice you will not get if you fall asleep.

Do not use an alarm clock to signal the end of your session. When you think the time is up, open your eyes and check the clock or your watch. End the session by slowly rousing yourself, moving your arms and legs as you get ready to continue your day.

If any of the relaxation techniques in this chapter or other chapters cause you pain or discomfort, talk with your healthcare professional. It may be possible to modify these techniques so you can use them, or you may be advised to avoid certain techniques.

Progressive Muscle Relaxation

As you are sitting or lying comfortably, close your eyes. Take three deep breaths. Breathe in slowly, each time silently counting up to five as you do. Breathe out slowly, each time silently counting up to 10 as you do. Do not count too fast when you breathe in or out. Some people find that counting "one-one thousand, two-one thousand, three-one thousand," and so on helps them count at a good pace.

After breathing out your third deep breath, focus your attention on the muscles of your legs. Tense your leg muscles and hold the tension as you silently count to five. Again, do not count too fast. Then, gradually release the tension in your legs as you count to 10. Allow the muscles of your legs to slacken. Notice how your legs feel comfortably heavy as they become relaxed.

Now focus on the muscles of your arms. Close your hands into fists. As you tighten your fists, tighten the muscles of your arms. Hold that tension to the count of five before gradually releasing it as you count to 10. Feel how your arms seem to become comfortably heavy as the muscles become increasingly relaxed.

Next, tense your abdominal muscles. Hold the tension to the count of five. Then, as you gradually relax those muscles, count to 10 silently. Feel your abdominal muscles, and the back muscles that tightened when you tensed your abdomen, become limp.

Now, bring your attention to your neck, shoulders, and upper back. Tilt your head back, pull your shoulders up and back, and hold the tension to the count of five. Release that tension as you slowly count to 10. Notice how these muscles feel as they loosen and become comfortably relaxed as you count.

Consider your face muscles next. Tense these by shutting your eyes more tightly, clenching your teeth, and tightly pursing your lips—all at the same time.

Count to five as you hold the tension in your facial muscles, then count to 10 as you release the tension.

Continue releasing the tension from your body. If you feel tension in your lower back, let it go. If you feel tension in your shoulders, neck, or jaw, let it go. Each time you exhale, let go of a little more tension. As you do this, you may become aware of the weight of your body as it is supported by the surface on which you are sitting or lying down (your chair, bed, or couch, for example). Notice the feelings associated with being relaxed, and with each breath allow yourself to become more deeply relaxed.

Sometimes as people become deeply relaxed, a set of muscles will, for an instant, jerk on its own. This is usually just a sign of being very, very relaxed. If it happens to you, it is likely to be an indication of how well you are doing.

Some people begin to feel anxious as they practice relaxation techniques. They report feeling that they are losing control. If this happens, it may be helpful to show yourself that the process of relaxing is really under your control. At any time during your practice, you can open your eyes and then close them again to continue becoming as relaxed as you prefer. You can also choose to end your relaxation session at any time. Making these choices as you practice the relaxation techniques allows you to gradually increase the benefits you receive. See Handout 2.5 for a quick guide to progressive muscle relaxation.

Summary

Chapter 2 covered approaches to encouraging the positive behavior of those to whom we provide care. The chapter made five main points regarding behavior. First, encouraging, triggering, and reinforcing positive behavior are the best ways to reduce or eliminate difficult behavior. The more often a person is doing positive things, the less likely it is that he or she will engage in challenging behaviors.

Second, promoting positive behavior is a more effective way to reduce challenging behavior than reprimanding, arguing, withholding privileges, or doing anything that the individual would experience as punishment. Punishment can often increase challenging behavior by intensifying the agitation, confusion, isolation, or self-doubt the person in need of care feels.

Third, three useful approaches to encouraging positive behavior are using active listening; allowing choices; and using praise, compliments, and acknowledgment. Active listening encourages the positive behavior of expressing thoughts and feelings in words and other positive behaviors. Allowing choices encourages both independence and cooperation. Using praise, compliments, and acknowledgment shows those we care for that they have value and reinforces positive behaviors.

Fourth, approaches for fostering positive behavior are more likely to cause someone who depends on your care to value his or her relationship with you. Valued relationships can promote a wide range of positive behaviors.

Fifth, avoid nagging, arguing, making repeated demands, threatening, or retaliating against someone who behaves in difficult ways. Generally, avoid negative responses to challenging behaviors. It is important to use positive approaches and avoid negative responses to difficult behavior with all care recipients, but especially with those who often behave in difficult ways.

Chapter 2 also expanded on the importance of stress management in effectively addressing difficult care situations. In particular, the chapter described the technique of progressive muscle relaxation.

Active Listening

Using active listening can provide needed emotional support for those in our care. It can help increase positive behaviors and decrease difficult behaviors.

Active listening techniques:

- Show the person that you are listening. Stop anything else you are doing. Make eye contact (as much as the person is able to tolerate). Show that you are paying attention by nodding your head or saying "Hmm," "Uh-huh," and "Oh."

- Listen to what the person says and what the person communicates nonverbally. Accept whatever feelings are presented. Avoid trying to correct the person's point of view.

- Restate in your own words what the person seems to be expressing through words or actions. As you listen, occasionally summarize the most important part of what the person has just said. Name the feelings that the person has expressed. Restate the reasons that the person believes are behind these feelings.

- Make suggestions, give advice, reassure, or offer a different perspective only after engaging in active listening—if at all.

Use active listening often. It can be helpful with all of those who depend on our care, especially those who are agitated, confused, or depressed.

Allowing Choices

Allowing care recipients to make choices can encourage positive behaviors. It is important to support decision making when care recipients are interested and capable of making choices.

Open-ended questions can help encourage capable and interested individuals to make decisions regarding their treatment, including the care and assistance they receive with activities of daily living, such as bathing, eating, and dressing. Unlike either-or and yes-or-no questions, open-ended questions do not have set answers.

Examples of open-ended questions:

- "When would you like to get out of bed today?"

- "When would you like to take your shower?"

- "What would you like to wear today?"

- "What time would you like to go to bed tonight?"

Limited-choice questions (Yes-and-no and either-or questions) can provide encouragement for people who are less capable or cooperative with necessary care because of confusion or bad moods. They are also helpful when the only choices you can offer are limited. These questions can often encourage positive, cooperative behaviors.

Examples of limited-choice questions:

- "May I help you with your lunch tray?"

- "Would you like me to help you out of bed now or when I can come back in 30 minutes?"

- "Would you like to take your shower this morning, or will you take it tomorrow?"

- "Which would you like to wear, the blue shirt or the green shirt?"

- "You can be the first or the third person I help to bed tonight. Which would you prefer?"

Very confused or overly stressed people might not make decisions well or may not understand the choices given to them. They may get agitated when given more choices than they can deal with, so it can be helpful to give simple step-by-step explanations of what you are doing and what you need the person to do. For example, you might say, "I'll help you put on your shirt. Here we go. Now, put this arm through this sleeve. Very good." It is important to praise effort and participation to reassure and encourage the person.

Using Praise, Compliments, and Acknowledgment

Praising or complimenting specific behaviors of those in our care can encourage and reinforce those behaviors. This makes those behaviors more likely to happen again.

Praising, complimenting, and acknowledging positive behaviors are usually good social reinforcers of behavior. Social reinforcers are typically the best kind of reinforcers.

Reinforcing positive behaviors is the best way to reduce challenging behaviors.

Remember to praise, compliment, and acknowledge positive things that care recipients do (particularly those who commonly engage in challenging behaviors). Make at least four positive comments for every one negative comment (about something that a resident should stop doing, for example).

In addition to praise and compliments, use nonverbal reinforcers, such as the following:

Smiles	Thumbs-up signs
Nods of approval or acknowledgment	Pats on the back
Hugs	Winks

Remember to praise, compliment, and acknowledge efforts and partial successes at positive, helpful, appropriate, independent, or cooperative behaviors. This can be especially important with people who frequently behave in difficult ways.

Be on the lookout for care recipients behaving in positive ways, and praise, compliment, or acknowledge what they are doing often.

Things to Avoid When Trying to Encourage Positive Behavior

When trying to reduce, eliminate, or prevent a challenging behavior, it is important to avoid the following:

- Nagging

- Arguing

- Repeatedly demanding that the person do (or not do) something

- Making threats (for example, "If you don't stop asking me for a cigarette, you won't get one" or "If you don't stop talking to me that way, you won't get out of bed")

- Giving the person a "dose of his or her own medicine" (for example, insulting someone who insults you)

- Withholding privileges

- Ignoring the individual

- Scolding or reprimanding

- Using punishment

- Defensively insisting that things are not the way the person sees them

- Laughing at the care recipient by making him or her the butt of jokes

- Engaging in power struggles

- Showing annoyance, frustration, or anger

These actions are not typically effective responses to challenging behaviors. Rather, they often trigger or reinforce challenging behaviors.

Progressive Muscle Relaxation

Spending 10–20 minutes per day clearing your mind and releasing tension from your body is an excellent method of managing the negative effects of stress on your mental and physical health and on your relationships with others. The following steps for progressive muscle relaxation can help. *If this or any other relaxation technique causes you discomfort or pain, stop and consult your healthcare professional for advice.*

1. **Pick a comfortable place** where you will not be disturbed for 10–20 minutes. Sit or lay down. Close your eyes.

2. **Take three slow, deep breaths.** As you breathe in, slowly and silently count to 5 (for example, "one one-thousand, two one-thousand . . ."). Then, slowly count to 10 as you exhale. For the rest of this exercise, breathe normally and naturally.

3. **Tense your leg muscles.** Then, slowly release the tension. You can do this step by pushing down with your legs to tense the muscles. Hold the tension until you do a slow, silent count to 5. Release the tension as you slowly count to 10.

4. **Tense and relax your arm muscles.** First, close your hands into fists. Tighten your fists. Push down with your arms. Feel the tension and hold it, counting slowly to 5. Then, release the tension gradually as you count to 10.

5. **Focus on your abdominal muscles.** Tighten those muscles. Hold the tension and count to 5. Release the tension to the count of 10.

6. **Tense the muscles of your neck, shoulders, and upper back.** Then, gradually release the tension. You can do this step by tilting your head back while pulling your shoulders up and back. Hold the tension to the count of 5. Release the tension while counting to 10.

7. **Focus on your face muscles.** Tense these muscles by shutting your eyes more tightly, clenching your teeth, and tightly pursing your lips—all at the same time. Hold the tension to the count of 5. Then, release the tension gradually as you count to 10.

After going through these seven steps, continue allowing tension to leave any muscles that are tight. Each time you exhale, let go of more tension and allow yourself to feel more relaxed.

(continued)

Progressive Muscle Relaxation

It is best not to fall asleep while you are practicing relaxation exercises. The goal is to become better at triggering and maintaining your body's ability to relax while you are awake.

Do not use an alarm clock to signal the end of your session. When you think the time is up, open your eyes and check. If the time is not up, close your eyes and continue your practice.

Sometimes people feel nervous that they will lose control when deeply relaxed. If this happens, open your eyes to show yourself that the process of relaxation is under your control. Then, gradually allow yourself to improve your body's ability to deeply relax.

EXERCISE 2.1

Think about an episode in which a person receiving care behaved in a way that was problematic. If you cannot think of an episode in which a care recipient engaged in a challenging behavior, think of one in which someone else did.

Briefly describe what the person was saying and how he or she was behaving.

Briefly describe the following:

1. How you used, or could have used, your body language to show the person that you were listening

2. How you restated, or could have restated, the meaning of the person's words or actions in your own words

3. How you named, or could have named, the emotion that the person was experiencing

4. How you restated, or could have restated, what the person believed were the reasons for his or her feelings

EXERCISE 2.2

Think of a time when you were providing care, therapy, or other services to someone. If you cannot think of such an example, think of a time when you were trying to get something done in some other way with another person.

Briefly describe what the two of you were doing.

Briefly describe the following:

1. How you gave, or could have given, the person choices by using open-ended questions

2. How you gave, or could have given, the person choices by using limited-choice questions

3. How you gave, or could have given, the person step-by-step explanations of what you were doing

EXERCISE 2.3

Think of a time when you were interacting with someone in your care, perhaps while providing care, therapy, or assistance, or while just passing him or her in the hall. If you cannot think of an example that involved someone in your care, choose an interaction you had with someone else.

Briefly describe the interaction.

Briefly describe the following:

1. Positive efforts the other person made during the interaction or at other times

2. Anything the person did during the interaction or at other times that was at least not negative

3. How you praised, complimented, or acknowledged—or could have praised, complimented, or acknowledged—those positive or neutral things. Remember that neutral behaviors can be considered progress toward more positive behaviors.

Finding Solutions to Challenging Behaviors

Chapter 2 demonstrated how our actions can encourage, trigger, or reinforce the positive behavior of those who depend on our care. This fact is related to another important point about behavior: Every behavior—good or bad—happens for a reason.

Chapter 3 explores methods of understanding behavior that can help us, and those in our care, find solutions to difficult behavior. This chapter describes the ABCs of Behavior method and cooperative problem-solving approach. It also explores "holding on," a strategy for containing our reactions to others' difficult behaviors. Chapter 3 also explains how to use mental imagery to reduce stress.

The Importance of Understanding Challenging Behaviors

Sometimes we make statements such as, "She hits people for no reason" or "His agitated behavior is unpredictable." These statements can be true in a certain sense. For example, we might mean that the hitting happens without what we consider to be acceptable justification, or that the occurrences of agitated behavior are difficult to understand and, therefore, also hard to predict.

As discussed in Chapter 2, using active listening often helps us find what prompts or reinforces challenging behaviors. By using active listening effectively, we can identify the thoughts and feelings that contribute to someone's behavior.

Containing our own thoughts and feelings as we interact with the person is also an important part of learning why an individual behaves in difficult ways. Understanding the person's thoughts and feelings allows us to adjust the environment in ways that convey our respect and concern. We can change the external influences contributing to the distress that typically underlies and fuels the difficult behavior.

External influences are often triggers and reinforcers of difficult behavior. For example, we might discover that instructing a resident to avoid talking in a despairing manner triggers his or her withdrawal into isolation and depression. We may also notice that as a consequence of the person's withdrawal, others do not interact as much with him or her, further reinforcing this individual's isolation, despair, and withdrawal. In this case, we can change the trigger that comes before the withdrawing behavior and the reinforcing consequence that follows it. For example, we could avoid saying, "Don't talk that way," and instead use active listening, changing what happens before the individual's isolating behavior (that is, changing the behavior's triggering antecedent). Then we could also alter the reinforcing consequence of the withdrawn behavior, perhaps by interacting with the person and continuing to use active listening.

The ABCs of Behavior and Interpersonal Interaction

The term *behavior trigger* means something that happened before a behavior—that is, an antecedent of the behavior. When we describe what happens in response to the behavior, we are talking about the consequence of the behavior. A consequence may reinforce the behavior, contributing to its continuing or becoming stronger.

The ABCs of Behavior concept can help us understand challenging behavior: There is at least one **A**ntecedent to each **B**ehavior, and a behavior that continues or gets stronger has at least one reinforcing **C**onsequence. The ABCs of Behavior, like active listening, is a useful tool for understanding some of the causes of behavior.

It is important to remember that no behavior is likely to have *only* internal or *only* external antecedents or consequences. It is often difficult for us to change internal causes of behavior. We cannot directly change past events that have led to someone's habits of behavior or lifelong ways of looking at things. We may have limited ability to modify a person's predisposition. There are some internal processes of mental and physical illnesses that we may not easily or quickly influence—and others that we may not be able to influence at all.

However, we can often have a direct, immediate influence on many of the external antecedents or consequences of a resident's behavior. First, we must determine which external antecedents may have triggered the behavior and identify which external consequences may have reinforced the behavior. The ABCs of Behavior approach helps us examine the process—or the context—in which a behavior happens. In reviewing this process, we often find previously unrecognized factors that have influenced a person's behavior. When we are aware of this pro-cess, we are typically able to modify it in ways that have a positive effect on the individual's behavior.

It is helpful to remember that how we interact with those in need of our care and attention is the most important source of reinforcement of their behaviors. In addition, our behavior may be a major source of triggering antecedents as well as reinforcing consequences. See Handout 3.1 for a review of the ABCs of Behavior approach.

Antecedents and Consequences

Mrs. Nicolls

Mrs. Nicolls was 69 years old. She used a wheelchair because she had difficulty walking and felt dizzy whenever she stood.

Felicity, a nursing assistant, was new to the long-term care community. She had never worked with Mrs. Nicolls before, but had heard others describe Mrs. Nicolls as "difficult." She heard that Mrs. Nicolls was uncooperative when being helped. Felicity's co-workers had also said that Mrs. Nicolls always accused people of taking her things, argued about everything, and remembered only what she wanted to remember. In addition, staff said that Mrs. Nicolls always hit others. However, whenever she was told that she should not hit others, Mrs. Nicolls said she never hit a soul. Finally, Mrs. Nicolls, who was Caucasian, was often described as a racist.

Felicity, who was an African American, was pleasantly surprised that Mrs. Nicolls was not very fussy with her. She was unsettled, however, to see Mrs. Nicolls hit others. This occurred each day after Mrs. Nicolls had finished lunch, just outside the dining room.

Because Mrs. Nicolls and many other residents who used wheelchairs moved slowly, there was usually a "traffic jam" of wheelchairs outside the dining room door. The residents bumped into each other, trying to make their way down that crowded section of the hallway. Very confused or frail residents would just sit in the way of the others.

Each day, Mrs. Nicolls was one of the first to leave the dining room, but she ended up in the middle of the traffic jam as others caught up to her and bumped into her wheelchair. After being bumped a few times, Mrs. Nicolls would curse and punch the next person who knocked into her. The more she got bumped, the louder she would curse and the more she would hit others. Some other residents cursed back at her, told her to stop, and even threatened to hit her back. Mrs. Nicolls only got more agitated, though, and she yelled and hit even more. At these times, she kept calling another resident, who was African American, a "f——— n———."

When staff told Mrs. Nicolls that her behavior was inappropriate, she just kept hitting other residents and yelling. The cursing and hitting only stopped when a staff member took Mrs. Nicolls out of the situation.

In a case like this, we can look for the antecedents and consequences that trigger and reinforce the challenging behavior. In this situation, Felicity decided to use the ABCs of Behavior to see what was triggering and reinforcing Mrs. Nicolls' agitated, hostile behavior. Felicity believed that the "A"—the antecedent—of the behavior was the overcrowded section of the hallway. This appeared to trigger the "B"—the behaviors—of cursing, yelling racist insults, and hitting others. Felicity noticed that the "C"—the consequence—of others yelling back, threatening, or telling Mrs. Nicolls that her behavior was inappropriate apparently reinforced her difficult behavior, making it continue and grow stronger. Felicity also noticed that the agitated behavior ended when the consequence of Mrs. Nicolls' behavior was she being wheeled out of the overcrowded situation. This consequence seemed to trigger calmer behavior from Mrs. Nicolls. In identifying these apparent triggers and reinforcers, Felicity was helped by keeping in mind that the most important triggers and reinforcers happen very close in time to the behavior. Usually, they come just before and right after the behavior starts.

Changing the Antecedents that Trigger the Problem Behavior

We can use what we learn about triggers or reinforcers to manage situations. This way we can help decrease how often or how long a behavior happens, or how intense the behavior is. We can also try to prevent situations that trigger the behavior.

After noticing the ABCs of Mrs. Nicolls' hitting, Felicity decided to watch Mrs. Nicolls whenever she began to leave the dining room after lunch. Felicity made sure to give Mrs. Nicolls help getting beyond the area that usually got "clogged." This changed what seemed to be the "A" of Mrs. Nicolls' agitated, hostile behavior. As a result, Mrs. Nicolls' hitting and shouting stopped.

When Felicity was not able to work with Mrs. Nicolls, she told the person who was going to be working with Mrs. Nicolls how she had been helping her avoid behaving in hostile, agitated ways. As other staff members increasingly followed Felicity's example, Mrs. Nicolls' challenging behavior dwindled and eventually stopped. In fact, staff members later recognized that the traffic jams were distressing to other residents, too. As a result, they ensured that there were no future traffic jams in the hallways.

Research conducted by psychologist Linda Teri and her colleagues has consistently demonstrated how helpful the ABCs of Behavior approach can be in cases such as Mrs. Nicolls', who had a diagnosis of probable Alzheimer's disease. It is important to note, though, that the basics of understanding triggers and reinforcers of behavior have been shown to be vital in understanding the behavior of people with a range of physical and mental health diagnoses, as well as people with no diagnosis at all.

Complete Exercise 3.1 for additional insight on the importance of identifying triggers and reinforcers.

Holding On: Dealing with Reactions to Challenging Behaviors

As mentioned previously, it can be difficult to deal with our feelings about a resident or about his or her challenging behavior. Yet, how we cope with these feelings can have a major influence on how successfully we address difficult behaviors.

In Mrs. Nicolls' case, Felicity felt initially unsettled, uncertain, and confused when she saw and heard her agitated, hostile behavior. Felicity's first reaction was anger. Then she thought, "This is not supposed to happen! This is just not supposed to happen! There is no excuse for violence or racism! Somebody should make her stop it!" Even though Mrs. Nicolls got along with Felicity, the hitting, cursing, and racial insults made her think that Mrs. Nicolls really was violent and racist. "Here it goes again," Felicity thought. "It's always the same. Racism and abusiveness that are always just under the surface come out one way or another, no matter what I do, no matter how well I do, or how helpful I am—no matter what anybody does. It will never stop." With these thoughts, her anger changed to a feeling of hopelessness.

At this point, Felicity thought she agreed with the others who said Mrs. Nicolls was difficult. Mrs. Nicolls' agitated, angry behavior contributed to Felicity's own initial reaction of anger and agitation. Fortunately, Felicity was better able to *hold on* and contain these feelings. She did not act on them. Unfortunately, part of what kept Felicity from acting at first was a sense of hopelessness. She believed that she could do nothing to change Mrs. Nicolls' behavior. She even started to feel helpless and worthless. This only went so far, though, before Felicity began to get angry again. She found herself thinking that no one had the right to make her feel this way, especially not Mrs. Nicolls. "I am not powerless, and I will not let anyone treat me like this," Felicity thought. She started to get fighting mad at the bumping and jostling that her sense of self always seemed to take.

Then Felicity realized with surprise how similar her own feelings and desired actions were to Mrs. Nicolls' behavior and apparent feelings when she got bumped and jostled in the hall. Felicity recognized that she was feeling empathy for Mrs. Nicolls because she understood that this was a very unpleasant experience for the woman. She saw that Mrs. Nicolls was not able to contain her feelings of anger in situations that overwhelmed her fragile abilities to cope. Felicity suspected that Mrs. Nicolls fought against feeling hopeless about her deteriorating physical and cognitive capabilities by fighting against others. Felicity thought, for example, that when Mrs. Nicolls treated her African American co-resident hatefully, Mrs. Nicolls was able to avoid focusing on what she hated about herself: her inability to get down the hallway and back to her room by herself and her view that she was nothing more than an obstacle, a hindrance.

It seemed to Felicity that if she acted on her own angry feelings toward Mrs. Nicolls—by reprimanding her, avoiding her, or withdrawing from her—she would probably reinforce Mrs. Nicolls' negative experience of herself. Felicity wanted to avoid this consequence. She suspected it would further motivate Mrs. Nicolls' difficult behavior.

While thinking all of this through, Felicity noticed that she was feeling less overwhelmed by her reactions to Mrs. Nicolls. She felt compassion for Mrs. Nicolls despite her actions and began to suspect there were ways to decrease Mrs. Nicolls' difficult behavior. In the end, using the ABCs of Behavior helped Felicity to no longer feel powerless when experiencing Mrs. Nicolls' agitated, hostile behavior. Furthermore, her work effectively solved a long-standing cause of resident distress in the long-term care community.

For a summary of the holding on approach, review Handout 3.2. Complete Exercise 3.2 to review how this strategy can be applied to your interactions with residents and others.

Ms. Oakley

Ms. Oakley was 75 years old and had been a resident of the long-term care community for about two years. Her left leg was amputated below the knee due to diabetes. She usually stayed in her room talking, sometimes shouting, to someone who was not there. Her words were hard to understand. Sometimes they sounded more like mumbling than actual words. When Ms. Oakley said words that were understandable, she did not put them into sentences that made sense to anyone. When the consulting psychiatrist visited and changed Ms. Oakley's medication, some of this behavior lessened. Still, Ms. Oakley kept to herself and said few understandable words other than "yes" or "no." Ms. Oakley only did tasks requested of her when she was asked to do them one at a time. Also, she did not change her clothing or wash herself, and she sometimes played with her excrement.

Miki, an LPN, was in the break room when Julio, a housekeeper, came in for some coffee. Miki looked pretty angry. Julio asked, "How's it going?"

"How's it going?! How's it going?!" she said, looking like she was trying not to explode. "She hit me! Oakley hit me! I hate this place!"

"Were you hurt?" Julio asked.

"This place is just too much!" Miki continued. "I don't come to work to be anybody's punching bag! She did it for no reason! I don't care how sick she is! She has no right to hit me!"

"You're pretty furious," Julio responded.

Miki went on, "It's always the same! You just do your best and where does it get you?! I don't have to take this abuse!"

"It's hard to go on doing your job when you get hit," Julio said.

"It is," Miki responded. "How can anyone be expected to work in a place like this? I just don't get it." Although still very angry, Miki was a bit calmer now.

"Did you report the incident?" asked Julio.

"Oh, yeah. I did the paperwork and all. I was told a psychiatrist will come over to see about adjusting Oakley's medication."

"You're not hurt?" Julio asked again.

"No. Just good and fed up," Miki answered.

"Want some coffee?" Julio asked.

"No, thanks, I don't need anything else revving me up just yet," Miki said. By this point, she was notably less upset.

Julio and Miki sat quietly for a while.

After a few moments, Miki said, "I was walking past her room and I looked in. She was sitting on the floor with her dress up and her diaper undone. She had poop on her hand and was chuckling while she reached up and smeared it on the bedspread. You know she does that kind of thing any chance she gets. Usually we're able to get to her to keep her clean. But over the past few days, because of the bad weather, people who are scheduled to work aren't getting in. And other people are away on vacation."

"Yeah, tell me about it. Everything that needs to be done can't be done quickly enough. It's been impossible," responded Julio.

"It is. It really is impossible," Miki added. "So when I saw what Oakley was doing, I rushed in to stop her from making more of a mess. I yelled, 'What are you doing? Stop that! Now I have to clean all of this up, and I don't have time for this!' She looked pretty surprised. And when I grabbed her arm to make her stop, she yanked her arm out of my hand and started swinging at me. I kept telling her to stop hitting me and that her behavior wouldn't be tolerated. But she just kept trying to hit me. It was a good thing that the new charge nurse, Joan, came in. Joan said she'd take care of it. She let me go finish helping the people I was supposed to shower so I could then give out meds."

It can be difficult in the heat of a moment to hold on, contain our feelings, and use the ABCs of Behavior. Sometimes we need time to step back, calm down, and look at what happened. For Miki, taking time off in the break room was a good idea. It also helped that Julio, someone she knew and felt comfortable with, made himself available through active listening. Although it is important for us to provide residents with emotional support through active listening, it is also important for us to provide it for each other. The more effectively we support each other, the less job stress and burnout we will feel.

When we are calmer, we can then use the ABCs of Behavior to understand what happened. Writing down our observations at this point may help us identify the likely triggers and reinforcers of a difficult behavior. Doing this can give us a better idea of how to prevent triggering and reinforcing the behavior in the future. For a guide to recording your observations, see the ABCs of Behavior Observation Form in the appendix. You can photocopy it and use it to record your observations when trying to help someone you provide care to reduce or eliminate a problem behavior.

If Miki had chosen to write down the ABCs of Ms. Oakley's hitting to understand the behavior better, she might have written what is shown in the sample that follows.

A Antecedent	B Behavior	C Consequence
I loudly told Ms. Oakley to stop what she was doing. I tried to stop her by holding her arm.	Ms. Oakley hit me. She repeatedly struck out at me.	I kept telling Ms. Oakley that her behavior would not be tolerated. I kept trying to restrain her arm.

Writing out the ABCs of Ms. Oakley's behavior might have helped Miki see the behavior as part of an interaction. It might have given Miki a chance to think of ways to change her behavior in future interactions to have a more positive effect on Ms. Oakley's behavior. Try completing Exercise 3.3 to see how the ABCs of Behavior can apply to someone in your care.

Beyond the Interaction

Miki and Julio's discussion showed how things outside the direct interaction between Miki and Ms. Oakley contributed to the incident. Miki was feeling overwhelmed by the amount of work she needed to do to make up for absent staff members. It is hard to be at our best under such circumstances. When we are stressed by too many responsibilities, we lose the patience needed to provide the best care to residents who have particularly difficult impairments.

Miki struggled with feeling powerless and angry. She had less success at holding on and containing those feelings than Felicity did during her work with Mrs. Nicolls. Miki acted on her anger by trying to take control of Ms. Oakley. Fortunately, when staffing returned to adequate levels, Miki once again was able to deal effectively with Ms. Oakley.

More About the ABCs of Behavior

When using the ABCs of Behavior, it is important to remember a couple of other tips to make it likely that your efforts will be successful. First, it is important to deal with only one or two challenging behaviors at a time. Do not try to solve all of a person's behavior issues at the same time. Second, to understand the ABCs of a particular behavior, stay focused on the situations in which the behavior happens. Use the ABCs of Behavior Observation Form in the appendix to record what happens to or around the resident before and after the behavior occurs. For difficult behaviors that happen frequently, triggering antecedents and reinforcing consequences may be found quickly, perhaps in a few days. For challenging behaviors that do not happen frequently, it could take two weeks or longer to find the antecedents or consequences. The following is another case example of how to use the ABCs of Behavior.

Mr. Youngquist

Mr. Youngquist was 70 years old. He was not able to use his right arm, hand, or leg because of a stroke. This affected his ability to perform certain activities, particularly because he was right-handed. However, psychological tests indicated that Mr. Youngquist's thinking and ability to understand others were not affected by the stroke. Still, he often had difficulty finding the words he wanted to say.

Maureen, a nursing assistant, was scheduled to work with Mr. Youngquist. Whenever she helped him into his pajamas at bedtime, the same embarrassing thing happened. One way or another, he would cup her breast with his hand or grab her bottom. When she told him to stop, he said, with some effort, "You . . . know . . . I . . . you like it." Despite her embarrassment, Maureen eventually told her supervisor, Barbara, who was also the charge nurse. When Barbara spoke with Mr. Youngquist about this behavior, he said, making an effort to speak clearly, that he had never touched Maureen that way. He said that Maureen must have misunderstood his accidentally touching her while she was helping him. Barbara still responded by emphasizing that such behavior was inappropriate and would not be tolerated.

Maureen had hoped that the behavior would stop after someone with as much authority as her supervisor talked to Mr. Youngquist, but it did not. The next day it happened again.

Later that day, Barbara checked with Maureen to see how things were going. When Maureen said that the problem was continuing, Barbara sympathized with her. Maureen could see that the sympathy was genuine. She understood Barbara's explanation that there were no further options for forcing Mr. Youngquist to stop his unwanted behavior other than filing formal legal charges. He could not even be discharged because his condition required skilled nursing care and his behavior would prevent any other long-term care community from admitting him.

Barbara asked Maureen if the problem was so difficult that she could no longer work with Mr. Youngquist. Barbara also asked if Maureen felt abused by Mr. Youngquist or by the way in which the situation was being handled. Maureen said she did not feel abused by Mr. Youngquist because she did not feel threatened by him or his behavior. Instead, she just felt annoyed when he fondled her. She also stated that she did not feel abused by the way the situation was being handled. In fact, she appreciated Barbara's concern and support. Maureen added that the problem was not significant enough to stop her from working with Mr. Youngquist. She really did like him—even if he could be annoying—and felt sorry for the upheaval in his life following his stroke.

Barbara asked Maureen what she thought should be done. Because Maureen had recently received some training on the ABCs of Behavior, she said that she would like to try this approach. She figured that if she could get an idea of what was triggering or reinforcing Mr. Youngquist's sexual behavior, she might be able to do something about it.

Barbara, who was familiar with the ABCs of Behavior approach, agreed that giving it a try was a good idea. She asked Maureen what she thought the ABCs were in regard to Mr. Youngquist's difficult behavior. Maureen believed that a possible trigger could be that he was a man, and that he might view women as sex objects. She guessed that Mr. Youngquist acted this way to assert that he was still a man despite the damage the stroke had done to his body.

Barbara said that all of that might be true. However, she added, Mr. Youngquist's lifelong attitudes about women were not likely to change quickly enough to prevent Maureen from being groped, and it was impossible to do anything about his being a man. Barbara pointed out, though, that changing these things was not necessary. The ABCs of Behavior focus on what occurred just before a behavior happened to see which specific factors triggered the behavior. The approach also looks at what happens in response to the behavior that may reinforce it.

Barbara suggested that Maureen use five questions to get an idea of the antecedents and consequences that might trigger and reinforce Mr. Youngquist's difficult behavior. She also asked Maureen to use these questions to record the apparent ABCs of Mr. Youngquist's behavior. The five questions were as follows:

1. When did the behavior happen—that is, at what time and on which day(s)?

2. At what location did the problem behavior happen? Describe the setting (private, crowded, loud, quiet, busy, not much activity, well-lit, dim).

3. What was happening to or around the resident when the behavior occurred?

4. Who was interacting with the resident when the behavior happened?

5. What did the person interacting with the resident do just before the behavior started and right after it began?

(See Handout 3.3 for a list of these questions.)

Maureen gave these answers:

1. It happened in the evenings between 8:00 and 10:00 P.M., every evening that I worked with Mr. Youngquist.

2. It only happened in Mr. Youngquist's room. It was private and quiet with the curtain drawn around his bed, and the door to the room closed. No one else was in the room.

3. I was helping Mr. Youngquist to change and get into bed.

4. I was interacting with Mr. Youngquist when the challenging behavior happened.

5. Mr. Youngquist grabbed my breast or bottom whenever I helped him change into his pajamas and get into bed. I told him, "Please stop touching me that way."

Maureen then used her answers to the questions to record the possible ABCs of Behavior for Mr. Youngquist (see the sample that follows).

A Antecedent	B Behavior	C Consequence
In the quiet privacy of his room, I helped Mr. Youngquist change and get into bed.	Mr. Youngquist cupped my breast or bottom with his hand.	I told him, "Please stop touching me that way."

Looking at what she wrote, Maureen could not see anything that she did not already know. Writing the answers to the questions and filling out the observation form did not seem to help her address Mr. Youngquist's behavior.

Barbara suggested that Maureen start by changing what would happen if Mr. Youngquist groped her again—changing the Consequence. Maureen had been asking Mr. Youngquist to stop touching her that way. Then she would continue helping him get ready for bed. Barbara proposed that Maureen let Mr. Youngquist know there would be a different consequence if he groped her again. Barbara explained that Maureen could say something like, "Mr. Youngquist, you have a choice. While I help you get to bed, you can either keep your hands to yourself or I will stop helping you. I'll stop what I am doing with you and leave you to yourself for about 15 minutes. Then, either I or someone else will come in to try to help you. If you touch any private part of my body, I will know you have chosen for me to leave you on your own for a little while." Barbara assured Maureen that this would be perfectly fine to do as long as leaving Mr. Youngquist did not put him—or anyone else—at immediate risk of harm. Barbara pointed out that by saying this as she went into Mr. Youngquist's room, Maureen would also be changing what usually happened before his troublesome behavior—that is, changing the Antecedents.

Barbara also asked Maureen to complete an ABCs of Behavior Observation Form to track Mr. Youngquist's groping behavior each day for the next week. Because the form contains space for three days, Maureen would need to make two copies of it to have space for each of the 5 days she would be working that week. Barbara suggested that Maureen keep using the five questions to help her complete the form. Maureen agreed to follow this suggestion.

That week, however, Maureen found it hard to be assertive in her interactions with Mr. Youngquist and did not tell him that she would leave him alone for 15 minutes if he touched her inappropriately. At the end of the week, Maureen explained this to Barbara but noted that she did complete the ABCs of Behavior Observation Form each day. Barbara said that she hoped Maureen could work on setting limits on what she would tolerate from Mr. Youngquist, and she asked to review the observation forms with Maureen (see the sample forms that follow).

ABCs of Behavior Observation Form

Date: 12/6/13   Time: 8:55 P.M.

A Antecedent	B Behavior	C Consequence
In the quiet privacy of his room, I helped Mr. Youngquist change and get into bed.	Mr. Youngquist cupped my breast or bottom with his hand.	I told him, "Please stop touching me that way."

Date: 12/7/13   Time: 9:35 P.M.

A Antecedent	B Behavior	C Consequence
In the quiet privacy of his room, I helped Mr. Youngquist change and get into bed.	Mr. Youngquist cupped my breast or bottom with his hand.	I told him, "Please stop touching me that way."

Date:____12/8/13_____   Time:_____9:45 P.M._____

A Antecedent	B Behavior	C Consequence
In the quiet privacy of his room, I helped Mr. Youngquist change and get into bed.	Mr. Youngquist cupped my breast or bottom with his hand.	I told him, "Please stop touching me that way."

Date:____12/9/13_____   Time:_____

A Antecedent	B Behavior	C Consequence
	The problem behavior did not happen today.	

Date:____12/10/13_____   Time:_____9:00 P.M._____

A Antecedent	B Behavior	C Consequence
In the quiet privacy of his room, I helped Mr. Youngquist change and get into bed.	Mr. Youngquist cupped my breast or bottom with his hand.	I told him, "Please stop touching me that way."

Date:____N/A_____   Time:_____N/A_____

A Antecedent	B Behavior	C Consequence
	N/A End of week	

Reviewing Observation Forms

Maureen said that except for the fourth day, the behavior happened consistently. Maureen explained that on the fourth day, Mr. Youngquist agreed to go to bed a little earlier so Maureen could help out with a resident who needed to be transferred to the hospital that evening. While Maureen was helping Mr. Youngquist, Carla, an LPN, knocked on the door and came in with his medications. Maureen had just drawn the curtain around the bed. Carla asked if she could help out, and both Mr. Youngquist and Maureen accepted her assistance. That evening, Mr. Youngquist did not engage in the problematic behavior.

Barbara asked what Maureen thought about the different conditions on the fourth night. Maureen thought that not having the usual amount of privacy might have prevented Mr. Youngquist from groping her. It seemed that privacy was an important triggering antecedent for Mr. Youngquist's unwelcome behavior. Barbara agreed with this hunch.

Barbara suggested that she would schedule someone to assist Maureen with changing and helping Mr. Youngquist to bed each night for the next week. She thought this might prove whether having another person in the room would help prevent Mr. Younquist's fondling behavior. Maureen liked this plan.

Remembering to Encourage Positive Behavior

Maureen also remembered that the best way to reduce or eliminate a challenging behavior is to encourage, trigger, and reinforce positive behavior. She realized that it was important for her and other staff members to encourage Mr. Youngquist's positive behaviors. Maureen decided to give Mr. Youngquist more positive attention, compliments, praise, and other social reinforcers for his efforts and successes at physical rehabilitation and for small steps toward self-care while she helped him change and get into bed. To Maureen, his inappropriate behavior signaled his need to feel potent, capable of pleasing and receiving affection. He wanted to feel he was accepted as a person, and as a man, Maureen believed. She thought he needed to feel valued and know that his affection had meaning—even if some of his ways of trying to achieve these things were not very skillful. Aside from the groping behavior, Mr. Youngquist usually was cooperative, friendly, and considerate; it appeared that he really was fond of her, Maureen believed.

Since he was regaining his ability to use language, encouraging Mr. Youngquist to express himself in words rather than inappropriate actions seemed a good idea to Maureen. Because active listening includes paying attention to nonverbal communication and restating or rephrasing what you think the person is expressing, Maureen decided it might be helpful to respond to Mr. Youngquist's attempts to touch her with active listening. This approach might encourage Mr. Youngquist's positive behavior of trying to use words rather than unwelcome actions to express himself. This would also change the Consequence of the behavior (Maureen saying, "Please stop . . . "). In fact, because the challenging behavior continued after this consequence, it most likely reinforced the behavior in some way. Maureen wondered if perhaps the consequence was a reinforcer because it was delivered in a way that suggested her underlying respect for, appreciation of, and interest in Mr. Youngquist.

Maureen decided to avoid Mr. Younquist's hand or gently redirect it while restating what his behavior seemed to mean and suggested about his feelings. Maureen thought she would say, "It is important to you to feel appreciated and valued, and you want me to feel that way, too," "You need me to know you like me. And it's important to you to know I like you," or, "You want to show me I'm important to you and you want to feel important to me." Maureen thought it might help to clearly state her preference for other expressions of his warm feelings, perhaps by saying, "I'm glad that you like me, but it's not polite for you to touch me that way. Not touching me that way and being your usual friendly, cooperative, considerate self would be a nice way to show me you like me. You could also try to use words and tell me what I do that you like. And I guess I could also tell you a bit more about what you do that I like."

Results

A co-worker assisted Maureen with Mr. Youngquist, as planned. Maureen and other staff members increasingly used social reinforcers to encourage his positive behaviors. As a result, Mr. Youngquist did not try to touch Maureen inappropriately again. Then, after several weeks of following the plan, unexpected staffing problems meant that Maureen ended up alone while helping Mr. Youngquist. She continued the positive comments and praise for his efforts in changing and getting to bed. When he seemed frustrated by difficulty in doing things or expressing himself, she used active listening. Mr. Youngquist did not touch her inappropriately. When Maureen spoke to Barbara about this development, they decided that Maureen could "go solo" with Mr. Youngquist again the next evening. That second evening was successful also. Maureen continued to use social reinforcers and active listening, and Mr. Youngquist did not engage in the challenging behavior. The third evening was the same, so Maureen and Barbara decided Maureen would continue to "go solo" with Mr. Youngquist. If the difficult behavior came back, they could always repeat the successful steps that they had used before:

1. Use the ABCs of Behavior to carefully observe the behavior, and identify its triggers and reinforcers.

2. Change the possible triggers or reinforcers, or both.

3. Encourage positive behaviors by frequently using praise, compliments, active listening, and other social reinforcers.

Try completing Exercise 3.4 to review how the ABCs of Behavior are important for uncovering triggers and reinforcers.

Mr. Fenety

Mr. Fenety was 44 years old. Before being admitted to the long-term care community, he had experienced long-time addiction to heroin. He had used other drugs, too—anything that would get him high. Mr. Fenety had received medical treatment for several overdoses. The last time he overdosed he was found unresponsive, without a heartbeat. Paramedics got his heart started again, but he had brain damage. The damage affected his sense of balance so severely that he had to rely on a wheelchair to get around. It also made his movements imprecise and jerky, which made it impossible for him to eat or dress on his own.

Mr. Fenety often pressed the call button to ask when he was going to get his medication, even though his memory was apparently not affected by his brain damage. Frequently, he sat in the doorway of his room calling, "Nurse . . . nurse . . . nurse." When someone attended to him, he would say that he did not feel well but would not give any specific details about his pain or discomfort.

In general, staff described Mr. Fenety as a demanding resident who was always complaining and insulting others. Mr. Fenety often screamed at staff, saying things such as, "Nobody around here does what they're supposed to do! I always have to tell everybody that I need things—they should know! You people don't know your jobs! You idiots are supposed to take care of me! I'll get your a—es fired!" According to information in his chart, Mr. Fenety had always behaved this way. Most staff members believed nothing would ever change that.

Kay, a registered nurse (RN) who was a charge nurse, noticed that when certain staff members responded to Mr. Fenety's calls for assistance, he whined about how nobody cared about him but did not scream at them. When other staff members, including Kay, told Mr. Fenety he would have to wait, he was more likely to scream demands, insults, or threats.

Kay explained to Mr. Fenety that his frequent calling and his screaming were disruptive and inappropriate. She told him that he would have to be more patient. If he called, someone would come to him as soon as possible, but if he was calling for something that was not critically important, he might have to wait until other priorities were met. Mr. Fenety replied, "Get the hell outta here, b——." Kay shook her head and left.

Kay told staff she was concerned that quickly responding to Mr. Fenety when he called for no reason only rewarded his demands for attention. She explained that they would address Mr. Fenety's challenging behavior by not giving him what he wanted when he wanted it when it was not immediately necessary for his care. The plan was to check on Mr. Fenety when he called, but then tell him he would be taken care of during routine care time if he did not need anything critically important. If he said anything insulting or screamed, he was to be told that his behavior was inappropriate. Staff members were then to tell him that they would return when his behavior improved.

Staff followed this plan for approximately a month. Unfortunately, Mr. Fenety's difficult behavior only worsened. Several times per day he had episodes of screaming insults, demands, and threats.

Kay talked with a charge nurse from another unit about the problem and was told about the ABCs of Behavior. She had trouble believing anything would help, especially considering Mr. Fenety's history of addiction and his apparently long-standing pattern of challenging behavior. Kay also thought that the existing behavior-modification plan was appropriate. If the current plan failed, then medication was the only option, Kay believed. However, the consulting psychiatrist was reluctant to use medication in this case. Unsure of what to do next, Kay decided to try using the ABCs of Behavior approach.

Determining Antecedents and Consequences

Kay thought about what usually happened just before one of Mr. Fenety's episodes. Typically, the antecedent ("A") seemed to be that he was not given immediate attention or was told to wait. The resulting behavior ("B") was that he screamed demands, insults, or threats. The usual consequence ("C") was that staff members told him his behavior was inappropriate and they would not help him until he stopped behaving abusively. Then they would leave him. Sometimes, though, staff had to provide the care necessary for Mr. Fenety's health and safety, such as changing a soiled undergarment or assisting when he fell down. In the end, Mr. Fenety got what staff thought he wanted—attention—even though it was only brief, negative, or necessary attention. It also seemed to Kay that the more negative attention Mr. Fenety received and the longer he was left to himself, the louder and more abusive his language became. So, the consequences—

negative attention, being left alone, and getting attention when it was absolutely necessary—seemed to be reinforcing Mr. Fenety's challenging behavior. Maureen then recorded the possible ABCs of Behavior for Mr. Fenety's verbal abuse (see the sample that follows).

A Antecedent	B Behavior	C Consequence
Mr. Fenety's call was not responded to as quickly as he wanted or he was told he would have to wait.	Mr. Fenety screamed demands, insults, or threats.	Mr. Fenety received negative attention, was left alone, or received brief attention when needed for health or safety.

Changing Antecedents and Consequences

Kay recognized that by trying not to reward Mr. Fenety's difficult behavior, the staff was focusing on only the consequence ("C") part of the ABCs of Behavior. It seemed that perhaps getting any attention—even negative attention—was reinforcing Mr. Fenety's unpleasant behavior. Also, giving periodic attention following his difficult behavior was sometimes unavoidable because care sometimes had to be provided to ensure that Mr. Fenety's health and safety were not at risk. Even if he was screaming, necessary care had to be provided.

Kay decided to experiment with changing the antecedent ("A") and consequence ("C"). She told the staff that she would try a new approach. That day, whenever Mr. Fenety called, she would try to get to him before he raised his voice. As she put this plan into action, Kay usually was able to get to Mr. Fenety before he engaged in challenging behavior. At these times, Mr. Fenety generally asked about when his medication or lunch would be coming, complained of some vague pain or discomfort, talked about what he did not like about other people, or talked about how no one seemed to care about him. Kay answered his questions and spent a minute or two using active listening. By responding to him in these ways, Kay changed the "A" to Mr. Fenety's verbal abuse, and when she responded in these ways, he did not scream demands, insults, or threats.

Whenever Kay was not able to get to Mr. Fenety before he started raising his voice, she ignored the difficult behavior and went to him anyway. Again, she usually spent a minute or two answering his questions and using active listening. By doing these things, Kay changed the "C" to his difficult behavior, and the episodes of the behavior were short and did not escalate.

During that day and the next one, Mr. Fenety raised his voice with Kay only two times per day. Previously, this behavior had been happening five or more times each day. When Mr. Fenety did raise his voice during Kay's experiment, it never reached the level of screaming. Mr. Fenety only threatened to get Kay fired once during the two days of Kay's experiment. Before she started the experiment, Mr. Fenety had made this threat at least five times every day.

It is good that Kay did not give up after the times Mr. Fenety did raise his voice or threaten her during her experiment. She had started to think, "What's the use? He's never going to change. Nothing works." Still, she stuck with her plan when she noticed that Mr. Fenety's unpleasant behaviors happened much less frequently than they had before she started her experiment. Kay learned that correcting antecedents and consequences leads to notable improvement of a challenging behavior.

Although Mr. Fenety's difficult behavior did not completely disappear, the improvement was encouraging. Kay spoke with the rest of the staff about the effective changes to their original plan. Now, Kay asked everyone to do what she had done during her experiment. When Mr. Fenety called, someone was to go to him before he raised his voice. Even if he did start to raise his voice, he was to be attended to anyway, and the tone of his voice ignored. His questions were to be answered, and his criticisms or complaints were to be responded to with active listening.

After two weeks of following the revised plan, Mr. Fenety never raised his voice with Kay. Other staff members reported that he rarely raised his voice with them, either. He shouted only seven times during the 2-week period. This was a major improvement because he had been screaming no less than five times a day before the change in the plan. In addition, the seven times that he did shout during the 2 weeks were the only times he threatened to get anyone fired. Kay and the rest of the staff had effectively helped Mr. Fenety with his negative behavior of screaming demands, insults, or threats.

Such dramatic change does not happen in all cases, usually because the antecedents or consequences are not managed as well as they need to be for improvement. In some cases, continued improvement is a satisfactory outcome. Also, in many cases, challenging behaviors return periodically. In any of these instances, we can use the ABCs of Behavior again. Those involved might more carefully look for correct "A's" and "C's" and then change the "A's," the "C's," or both the "A's" and the "C's." This concept is illustrated by the continuing case involving Mr. Fenety.

Kay was encouraged by Mr. Fenety's improvement, but she recognized that he still called for assistance more than any resident in his unit. The requests he made when he called were not about immediate threats to his or anyone else's well-being. They were typically about tasks that he was able to do himself or for information he probably already knew. Sometimes this behavior of frequently calling for assistance made it hard to respond to Mr. Fenety because Kay and other staff were busy with other residents. Other times, the behavior interfered with the staff's ability to respond quickly to other residents' needs. In addition, Mr. Fenety's behavior made it nearly impossible for staff to take a much-needed break. To address these issues, Kay had a conversation with Mr. Fenety.

"Please call for help only when you really need it," Kay began.

Mr. Fenety responded, "I don't see why I have to wait. I'm always the last one taken care of."

Kay said, "Mr. Fenety, you are not always the last one. What are we supposed to do—leave other residents who need us just to come and tell you what you already know, such as when your medication is coming?"

Mr. Fenety yelled, "I don't care about anyone else! I'm number one! Not you! Not anyone else!"

Kay saw that her direct confrontation of the problem was triggering Mr. Fenety's agitation, so she used active listening and said, "I guess you need to feel like you matter, like someone cares enough to treat you like you're number one." As she continued using active listening, Mr. Fenety quickly calmed down.

Trying to get Mr. Fenety to correct a behavior that he did not consider a problem was not the best approach. Kay wondered if using the ABCs of Behavior could help. The first step was to use the ABCs to look at Mr. Fenety's difficult behavior of frequently demanding attention (see the sample that follows).

A Antecedent	B Behavior	C Consequence
Mr. Fenety was alone in his room.	Mr. Fenety started pushing the call button or calling "Nurse . . . nurse . . . nurse."	A staff member went to Mr. Fenety.

Earlier experience with Mr. Fenety showed Kay that changing "C" could lead to increased problems. She and other staff members knew first-hand that ignoring Mr. Fenety triggered greater difficulty, with even more screaming of demands, threats, or insults. Going to Mr. Fenety triggered less problematic behavior. Rather than persistently screaming, he simply continued to call out or use the call button often. Although this was an improvement, going to Mr. Fenety after he called out or used the call button did reinforce that particular behavior.

Changing the Antecedent

Kay decided that it might be a good idea to try changing the antecedent to Mr. Fenety's challenging behavior of frequently calling for someone to attend to him. Because being alone in his room usually came before his calling for assistance, Kay guessed that being alone in his room was a trigger. Mr. Fenety rarely used the call bell or called out while others (visitors, other residents, staff, for example) were with him, and he did it most often in the evening until about 9:00 P.M., his bedtime.

Kay was working evenings, so she decided to try another experiment. Arriving at work each evening, the first thing she did was visit Mr. Fenety's room. She was usually able to do this before he called out or used the call bell. For a week, she also went to see Mr. Fenety every 20 minutes from after dinner until 9:00 P.M. It was difficult to do this because Kay had other responsibilities. However, a couple of staff members helped out enough that Kay had time to try her plan.

When she went into Mr. Fenety's room, Kay usually just asked how he was or engaged in small talk with him. Mr. Fenety still had a tendency to complain, so Kay used active listening with him often. Kay usually limited these visits to no more than 2 minutes. Sometimes Mr. Fenety asked Kay for help with activities that he was able to do independently. Kay noticed that although she helped in such instances, Mr. Fenety still did most other things he could do for himself. She and others had believed that helping Mr. Fenety, when he asked, with tasks he was able to do on his own would reinforce and increase his seeking help.

Kay's brief visits to Mr. Fenety's room seemed to work very well. During the first week of following this plan, Mr. Fenety called out or used the call bell much less frequently during the evenings. Previously, he engaged in this behavior eight or more times every evening. After Kay began her visits, Mr. Fenety never called more than twice in an evening. In fact, Mr. Fenety did not call out or use the call bell even once during the last two evenings of the week.

After Kay began following her plan, she did feel disappointed whenever Mr. Fenety called for assistance. However, she reminded herself that his behavior really had improved. This is an important point. Behavior change is often gradual. Also, challenging behavior occasionally increases when a resident feels stressed by a worsening physical condition, a move to a new room, a roommate dying, or other changes in routines or important relationships (changes in staff due to turnover or scheduling, for example). Behavior change is often not immediate or complete. It is important to recognize any improvements. Acknowledge your partial successes and those of the person in your care. They are steps along the way to the best possible outcome. See Handout 3.4 for a list of realistic and unrealistic goals regarding the improvement of challenging behaviors.

Continuing Success

Kay spoke with the rest of the staff about her findings. By the next week, it became routine for more staff to briefly but frequently shoot the breeze with Mr. Fenety. Staff members were typically able to stop by before he called out. Active listening was usually all he needed when he complained about his health or other people. When he asked for help, it was usually with a task that could be easily addressed and did not interfere with his ability to do things independently. By the end of the second week, Mr. Fenety's behavior had continued to improve. Most evenings he did not call out at all. When he did engage in this behavior, he only did so once or twice per evening.

As the other staff members helped out, Kay gradually cut back on her visits with Mr. Fenety. On the first night of the second week, she went to his room every 25 minutes. The next night she visited every 30 minutes. Kay decided that visiting Mr. Fenety every 30 minutes would not interfere with her other work or burden her.

Kay also realized that in the future other staff members could gradually increase the amount of time between their visits to Mr. Fenety. They could do this until they found the most workable balance between Mr. Fenety's need for social interaction and their need do other things.

Visiting Mr. Fenety before he called for assistance reinforced his behavior of quietly watching television, which is what he was usually doing when staff came to visit. The "B" in the ABCs of Mr. Fenety's evening behavior became "sitting quietly." The "C" became the social interaction of having staff visit, use active listening, chat, or respond to what was usually a small request for help. In this case, the "A" to Mr. Fenety's quiet behavior was his not being alone in his room for longer than he could tolerate. By gradually *stretching* the time between their visits to Mr. Fenety, staff members were also helping him to stretch his ability to tolerate being alone for slightly longer periods. The technique of stretching can be useful in working with residents who are demanding or frequently seek attention. See Handout 3.5 for an overview of this technique.

Cooperative Problem Solving with Care Recipients

As mentioned previously, the ABCs of Behavior approach is particularly helpful when a person does not realize or acknowledge that there is a problem or when the individual cannot change elements of the situations that trigger or reinforce the challenging behavior. However, in cases where the person is willing and able to be actively involved in finding a solution to the problem, we can use a different, cooperative problem-solving approach.

This problem-solving approach starts with the use of active listening to help us restate the individual's feelings and say in our own words what the individual seems to say is the problem. Next, we ask the person if there are times when the problem does not happen. If there are such times, we discuss what is happening at those times. This can give the individual a chance to think about and describe what can be done to adjust the problem situation. Together with the person we can consider which actions taken by the individual and by others contribute to preventing or eliminating the problem. If necessary or useful, we can also encourage the individual to reminisce about similar problems in his or her past. We can ask questions such as, "Have you always felt this frightened?" or "Have you never felt safe?" By including the words *always* and *never*, we may trigger a person's memories of how similar problems happened in the past, how they do not always happen, and how the resident previously coped with them.

Ms. Quigley

We met 77-year-old Ms. Quigley in Chapter 1. She had severe difficulty breathing, was very anxious, and often called for someone to come to her room. She called so frequently that it was difficult for staff to attend to her and accomplish their other responsibilities.

Peggy, a social worker, visited Ms. Quigley to see what could be done about these frequent calls for attention. When Ms. Quigley asked Peggy to take the cover off the lunch tray that was right in front of her, something Ms. Quigley was able to do herself, Peggy did it. When Ms. Quigley complained of how no one understood how sick she was and how much help she needed, Peggy used active listening. When Ms. Quigley spoke about her fear of being alone and her constant anxiety, Peggy continued using active listening.

Ms. Quigley still seemed nervous, her hands quickly moving among the plates and utensils on her tray without any apparent purpose other than to touch them or move them slightly one way and then another. However, she was noticeably less nervous than when Peggy had first walked into the room.

Peggy asked, "I know you were just saying that you always feel anxious, Ms. Quigley, but are there times when you feel more anxious and times when you feel a little less anxious?"

Ms. Quigley explained, "I feel less anxious now that you're here listening to me."

Peggy then asked, "Have you always had a problem with anxiety?"

Ms. Quigley responded, "I was high-strung from an early age. I used to deal with it by being active. I was always very social when I was young, going to parties and dances, spending time with my friends and on the telephone, and being involved in church activities."

"What has helped you since you haven't been able to be as active as you used to be?" Peggy asked.

Ms. Quigley said, "When I'm around other people, even if I'm just watching them as they walk past or do other things, I'm less anxious. Talking to someone who will really just listen is the most help."

Peggy and Ms. Quigley then spoke with the charge nurse. They arranged to have an oxygen tank put on Ms. Quigley's wheelchair and to let her spend time each day near the front door in the lobby, where she would see staff, visitors, and other residents coming and going. The plan included assistance in getting Ms. Quigley to the lobby. It also included two 15-minute visits per week from Peggy so Ms. Quigley could talk to someone who would "really just listen."

Mr. Dukmejian

Late one night in the long-term care community, 72-year-old Mr. Dukmejian threw a trash basket. It smashed against a wall in the hallway. This occurred after a couple of weeks during which he was increasingly active and noisy in his room at night, playing his radio loudly and singing. Ray, the new night charge nurse, went to talk with Mr. Dukmejian.

Mr. Dukmejian talked about needing to keep "those strange people" out of his room at night. Ray used active listening, rephrasing and restating what Mr. Dukmejian said, and commented that Mr. Dukmejian seemed frightened. Mr. Dukmejian continued by saying it really was not safe for him to go to sleep with people coming in to "go to the bathroom" on the floor in his room. He was afraid they would beat him up and have sex with him, he said. "And I'm not even gay," Mr. Dukmejian asserted.

"Are there times when they don't come into your room at night?" Ray asked.

Mr. Dukmejian pointed out, "They're not around now, while we're talking."

Ray asked, "Has nighttime always been frightening for you?"

Mr. Dukmejian explained, "When I was growing up, I shared a room with my older brothers. Then, after I got married, my wife and I shared the same bed for 50 years. So, no, I never was scared at night."

Ray commented, "Knowing there are people around that you feel safe with seems to help. What can you do when you wake up at night and do not feel safe?"

Mr. Dukmejian said he was not sure, so Ray suggested, "You seem to feel safe with me as we talk. If you wake up at night and feel frightened or if those people come back, maybe you could come sit near the nurses' station while I work."

Mr. Dukmejian replied, "That's a good idea."

Mr. Dukmejian and Ray worked together to resolve the problematic situation. See Handout 3.6 for a summary of this approach. Try completing Exercise 3.5 to learn more about personal applications of this method.

Coping with Stress by Using Mental Imagery

As already noted, how we cope with stress can have a significant impact on how we react to difficult behavior. This section of chapter 3 describes mental imagery and how it can be used to manage the stress we can feel.

Mental imagery can be used by itself or in combination with other relaxation techniques, such as progressive muscle relaxation. To use mental imagery, sit or lie comfortably in a spot where you will not be disturbed for 10–20 minutes. Imagine yourself in a pleasant, relaxing place. See, hear, feel, and smell the things that make it a peaceful place. See the colors and shapes of things and the gentle movements. Hear the sounds. Feel the comforting touch of a soft breeze, the "just right" temperature, or the sensation of your body being supported or perhaps even floating. Smell the fragrances.

For example, see yourself at the beach on a day when the temperature is comfortably warm. The sky is beautifully clear and blue, with occasional puffy white clouds that drift slowly over the ocean. There are a few people here and there, strolling or lying on the sand. A gentle, warm breeze brushes your face as you walk barefoot on the sand. You feel the sand massage your feet with each step that you take. The breeze has a clean, fresh, mildly salty fragrance. You stop walking, stretch out on the sand, and look up at a few clouds against the blue sky. The warm sand supports your body as it conforms to the contours of your back and your legs. Watching the clouds drift lazily by, you hear the distant, occasional sounds of children happily playing and a seagull's cry. As the sights, sounds, and scents of this place deepen your relaxation, feel the weight of your body against the sand get pleasantly heavier as you become more deeply relaxed.

Continue your relaxation session for the time you have set aside. When the time is up, gently stretch your arms, legs, and neck before going on with your day.

To review a step-by-step description of the mental imagery process, see Handout 3.7.

Summary

Chapter 3 discussed how both positive and negative behaviors happen for specific reasons. It also described ways of finding solutions to difficult behaviors. The first approach to finding solutions was the ABCs of Behavior method, which has the following elements:

A: Every behavior has at least one *antecedent*—an event, or thing that happens, that precedes it and serves as a trigger.

B: A *behavior* is any action.

C: If a behavior continues or gets stronger, at least one *consequence*, or event that comes after the behavior, is a reinforcer.

By carefully observing what happens before and after a behavior, we can find the likely triggering antecedents and reinforcing consequences that need to be changed in order for the behavior to change.

The second method of finding solutions to difficult behaviors is cooperative problem solving. The steps of the cooperative problem-solving method described are as follows:

1. Use active listening to get a clear idea of what the person engaging in a challenging behavior sees as the problematic situation.

2. Ask the person about what is happening when the problem is not present, if there are such times.

3. Ask the individual to reminisce about times in his or her life when the problem was prevented or coped with, and about how it was prevented or coped with.

4. Use the person's replies in Steps 2 and 3 to decide with him or her how to deal with current difficulties.

5. If the cooperative problem-solving method does not work, use the ABCs of Behavior approach.

Chapter 3 also described the technique of stretching. This technique is based on the ABCs of Behavior and can be very helpful for dealing with someone who is demanding or frequently engages in disruptive attention-seeking behavior. Stretching involves two steps. First, routinely go to the person *before* the difficult behavior occurs, ignore the behavior if it happens, respond to the person's request, and use praise and other social reinforcers for any behavior that is not a challenging behavior. Second, gradually increase the amount of time between routine visits to the individual to help stretch his or her ability to tolerate longer periods of times without being the focus of attention.

In addition, this chapter discussed setting realistic goals. We work toward realistic goals when we help someone decrease the frequency of a challenging behavior, the intensity of the behavior, or both. For some people, a reasonable goal may simply be that when episodes occur, they are briefer in duration. Remember that improvement is often gradual. In addition, it is best to work on reducing or eliminating only one or two challenging behaviors at a time.

This chapter also encouraged us to contain our own strong emotional reactions that can occur when we face care recipients' challenging behaviors. Such emotions often reflect the same feelings that overwhelm the people in need of care. By containing these feelings and modeling nonaggressive, helpful behaviors for those in our care, we shoulder some of the burden of their feelings and perhaps encourage them to engage in more positive behaviors.

Finally, Chapter 3 further explored the concept of addressing stress among caregivers using mental imagery.

The ABCs of Behavior

When dealing with a difficult behavior, remember to use the ABCs of Behavior:

A   Every behavior—positive or negative—is triggered by something. What happens just before a behavior that triggers the behavior is an **A**ntecedent of the behavior.

B   A **B**ehavior is any action. It can be good or bad, positive or negative.

C   If a behavior continues or gets stronger, what comes after the behavior—that is, the **C**onsequence of the behavior—is reinforcing the behavior.

No behavior is likely to be triggered and reinforced only by internal factors or only by external factors. We can usually have a direct, immediate effect on many external influences—changing external triggers and reinforcers of a difficult behavior. By doing this we can help reduce or even eliminate a challenging behavior.

It is important to look at what we and others do that may trigger or reinforce a care recipient's behavior. Other people—intentionally or not—are the most important sources of triggers and reinforcers of care recipients' behavior.

Holding On: Dealing with Reactions to Challenging Behaviors

First, when you have strong feelings about the behavior of a person in your care, hold on. Do not immediately react out of feelings such as anger, frustration, disgust, or hopelessness.

Second, ask yourself if your feelings resemble what the person in your care feels.

Third, think of what kind of behavior you would like to see from the person (for example, helpful, cooperative, nonaggressive, considerate).

Fourth, behave in the way you would like the individual to behave, even if he or she has behaved—or is behaving—in difficult ways.

Fifth, if the person's behavior does not become more positive, look for ways that your behavior (for example, acting defensive, annoyed, angry, impatient, hurt, or distant) could be triggering or reinforcing the difficult behavior.

Finally, consider changing those triggers or reinforcers.

Finding Triggers and Reinforcers of Challenging Behaviors

When we are trying to see what the triggering **A**ntecedents are to a challenging **B**ehavior, and trying to find the reinforcing **C**onsequences, the following five questions can be helpful:

1. When did the behavior happen—that is, at what time and on which day(s)?

2. At what location did the behavior happen? Describe the setting (private, crowded, loud, quiet, busy, not much activity, well-lit, dim).

3. What was happening around or to the person when the difficult behavior happened?

4. Who was interacting with the person when the behavior happened?

5. What did the person interacting with the care recipient do just before the challenging behavior started and right after it began?

Realistic Goals for Residents' Challenging Behaviors

We are likely to have unrealistic goals when we

- Expect challenging behaviors to never happen

- Expect a challenging behavior that happens frequently to go away immediately

- Expect a very intense challenging behavior to completely stop right away

- Consider challenging behaviors as simply wrong and not supposed to happen

We can develop realistic goals for helping residents change challenging behaviors when we

- Remember that challenging behaviors sometimes change gradually

- Remember to look for decreased frequency of challenging behaviors

- Remember to look for decreased intensity of challenging behaviors when they do occur

- Remember to look for shorter episodes of challenging behaviors

Having unrealistic goals can lead us to

- Believe that nothing works and that nothing will change

- Give up on effective ways of dealing with challenging behaviors

- Feel helpless, angry, and burned out

Having realistic goals can

- Help us stay focused on effective ways of dealing with challenging behaviors

Stretching

Stretching is a way of helping reduce demanding or disruptive attention-seeking behavior. It helps by gradually lengthening the amount of time a person can go without receiving attention for concerns that are not immediately critical for his or her health or well-being.

Step 1

A. Make it routine to go to the individual *before* he or she calls out, shouts, or makes demands. Initially, this might mean going to the person quite often.

B. Go regardless of whether you can reach the person before a demanding or attention-seeking behavior occurs.

C. If the individual makes a demand, respond as though the demand is a reasonable, polite request. Do what you can to respond to this request, assuming that doing so does not pose an immediate risk to the health or well-being of the person or anyone else.

D. If the individual complains, argues, hurls insults, or makes verbal threats, use active listening skills. In addition, use social reinforcers, such as praise, compliments, thumbs-up signs, pats on the back, or hugs, for *any* positive behavior.

Step 2

A. Once you establish a pattern of getting to the person *before* a demanding or disruptive attention-seeking behavior starts, you will probably see a decrease in the behavior within a few days. If there is no significant decrease after 2 weeks, it is likely that the person has not consistently been attended to *before* the negative behavior starts.

B. Once a pattern has been established and there has been a significant decrease in the challenging behavior, stay with the plan for 3–7 days. Then, begin gradually stretching the amount of time between your visits by a few minutes—probably by no more than 5 minutes at the beginning.

C. If the difficult behavior does not significantly increase after a day of stretching, the next day try stretching the time between visits by a few more minutes. Each day, gradually stretch the amount of time until you determine what length of time the person is currently able to tolerate.

(continued)

Stretching

D.   If the challenging behavior increases in frequency or severity, begin again with Step 1. This time, lengthen the amount of time between visits more gradually. Make the increases in the length of time between visits smaller. Wait 2 or more days before making further increases.

E.   If you try the stretching process twice and it does not help, try it again and watch carefully for triggers and reinforcers of the difficult behavior. Record your observations of what is happening to or around the resident before and after the behavior starts.

Cooperative Problem Solving

It is often helpful to encourage a care recipient's active involvement in resolving problems that trigger or reinforce challenging behaviors. Using the following five steps can foster cooperative problem solving with residents:

1. Use the active listening techniques of rephrasing or restating what the person seems to be saying verbally and nonverbally. Name his or her feelings to the degree that the individual can tolerate. Using these techniques can help us understand the problem from that person's perspective.

2. Ask the individual if there are times when what he or she considers to be the problem does not happen. What are the circumstances when the problem does not exist? What do others do that prevents or stops the problem? What does the individual do that prevents or stops the problem?

3. If needed or helpful, encourage the resident to think back on his or her life. Ask questions such as, "Have you always felt _____?," "Has it never been any different at any time in your life?," or "What helped when things such as this happened (or when you felt this way) in the past?"

4. Use the person's replies to Steps 2 and 3 to decide with him or her what to do in the current situation.

5. Sometimes the cooperative problem-solving method does not work. If the person does not or is not able to cooperate or if his or her behavior worsens during the cooperative problem-solving process, try to determine what might be triggering or reinforcing the behavior.

Mental Imagery

You can use this relaxation technique alone or in conjunction with other relaxation techniques. Remember, practicing relaxation techniques for 10–20 minutes per day can be very helpful in managing the negative effects of stress on your mental and physical health.

1. Sit or lie down in a comfortable position where you will not be disturbed for 10–20 minutes. Close your eyes and imagine yourself in a pleasant, relaxing place, such as a beach, a park, or a forest with a stream—any place that you find relaxing.

2. In your mind, focus on the details that make the scene you have chosen a comforting place. You might see the pleasant way the sunlight sparkles on water, the soft green of a patch of grass, or curtains stirred by a slight breeze.

3. Hear the relaxing sounds of the place you have in mind. They might be a light breeze rustling the uppermost leaves of the trees, birds singing, or the sounds of a meal being prepared in the kitchen.

4. Feel what is comforting about the place. You might feel the warmth of the sun, the weight of your body as you are stretched out in the grass, or the coziness of wearing a sweater.

5. Notice the fragrances. These might be the scent of fresh earth, flowers, or a favorite meal being made.

Become aware of the sights, sounds, and sensations that you find comforting about your peaceful, relaxing place. As you do, enjoy the experience of becoming more pleasantly at ease, calm, and relaxed.

EXERCISE 3.1

Think about a time when a recipient of your care behaved in a way that was problematic. If you cannot think of a time when a person receiving your care behaved in such a way, think about an incident in which someone else did.

Briefly describe the behavior.

Briefly describe the following:

1. Possible external triggers for the behavior (Remember that the most important triggers happen very close in time to the behavior, usually just before the difficult behavior starts.)

2. Possible external reinforcing consequences that might have contributed to the continuation or worsening of the behavior (Remember that reinforcing consequences usually happen very close in time to the behavior, usually right after the behavior starts.)

3. What you did, or could have done, to change what was happening in response to the behavior—that is, to change the reinforcing consequences

4. What you did, or could have done, to help prevent the person's difficult behavior from being triggered in the future

EXERCISE 3.2

Think of an incident in which someone in your care behaved in a difficult way. Think of an incident involving someone else if you cannot think of one involving a person receiving care from you.

Briefly describe the difficult behavior.

What emotion was the person probably experiencing?

Was your emotion at the time similar to what the other person seemed to be feeling? If not, think of a different incident—maybe one involving a different person—in which it is easier to see the similarity between the emotions both of you were feeling.

Describe the following:

1. How you would have liked the person to behave

2. The way you behaved, or could have behaved, to exemplify the type of behavior you would have liked the other person to display

EXERCISE 3.3

Think of a person in your care who engaged in a challenging behavior. If you cannot think of such a person who has behaved in a difficult way, think of someone else who has. Using the following directions, fill out the ABC box below for a particular incident.

First, under "B," record the challenging behavior. Be specific. For example, instead of saying, "She was aggressive," describe the action in which the person engaged, such as, "The resident screamed that I was lazy and stupid."

Next, under "A," record what was happening to or around the person immediately before the behavior began. Again, be specific. Instead of saying, "I was delivering care to her," it is more helpful to write something such as, "I told Mrs. X that I would help her out of bed in a little while after she said that she wanted to get out of bed."

Finally, under "C," record what happened immediately in response to the person's difficult behavior. Be specific. For example, rather than saying, "I reported the behavior to the charge nurse," it is better to say something such as, "I walked out of Mrs. X's room without saying anything to her."

Antecedent	Behavior	Consequence

EXERCISE 3.4

Photocopy the ABCs of Behavior Observation Form in the appendix. During the next week, use copies of the form to track one care recipient's challenging behavior that happens frequently (at least daily). If you cannot do this by observing a care recipient, do it by observing someone else. At the end of the week, determine which changes you would recommend in the antecedents or consequences (or both) of the behavior in order to help reduce or eliminate the challenging behavior. Record your recommendations in the space below.

EXERCISE 3.5

Think of an incident in which a resident engaged in a difficult behavior. If you cannot think of an incident involving a resident, think of one involving someone else.

Briefly describe the behavior.

Briefly describe the following:

1. How you used or could have used active listening and what the other person seemed to consider as the problem

2. How you asked or could have asked the person about times when the problematic situation does not happen

3. How you encouraged or could have encouraged the person to think of past experiences when the problem—as that person saw it—did not exist or when the problem was dealt with effectively

4. How you used or could have used the person's replies in Steps 2 and 3 to help reduce or eliminate his or her difficult behavior

5. What you did or might have done if cooperative problem-solving steps were not helpful with this person

CHAPTER 4

Stress and the Roles of Thinking and Feeling

One of the most important parts of effectively dealing with the challenging behaviors of those who depend upon us for care is coping with how we feel about what the care recipient does. The strength of what we feel affects how we react when a care recipient behaves in demanding, insulting, threatening, agitated, confused, or depressed ways. Some of the feelings we have while dealing with difficult behavior include frustration, anger, hopelessness, depression, confusion, and even fear. Such feelings, when they are strong or persistent, *are* the stress we feel. They can have a significant impact on our mental and physical health.

This book's techniques for helping reduce or eliminate challenging behaviors can help us manage stress. Often, knowing how to effectively handle a difficult situation can make the situation less stressful. The techniques in this book can also help by reducing or eliminating the situations that we find stressful. The stress management techniques throughout the book may help, too.

Being faced with challenging behaviors is common for caregivers. In some cases, reducing—not eliminating—a difficult behavior may be the only realistic short-term goal. The longer-term goal might be to further reduce the problem. On the way to our short-term and long-term goals, we need to cope with our own reactions to the difficult behavior. How we manage our reactions to the behavior can have a major impact on how reachable that goal is.

This chapter looks at how the relationship between thinking and feeling can be used to help us deal with the stress of working with those who need our close care and attention. In addition, the chapter further explores how our own feelings can provide clues for how to best respond to difficult behavior. Chapter 4 ends by describing another relaxation method to use during a quiet time in your day. This simple method for managing stress focuses on breathing to deepen relaxation.

Thinking and Feeling Explained

Thinking and feeling are connected: How we feel affects how we think, and how we think affects how we feel. The work of Nobel Prize–winning psychologist Daniel Kahneman and his colleagues has greatly furthered understanding of this link, particularly the role of emotion in influencing thinking. If we feel too frightened, anxious, angry, or excited, for example, our thinking can become inflexible, overly automatic, even confused. Also, if we frequently have thoughts such as, "I'm not good at anything. Nobody ever really cares about me," we are more likely to feel hopeless and depressed.

To deal effectively with stressful situations such as caring for someone who behaves in difficult ways, it is important for us to try to recognize and manage our own feelings and thoughts about what the care recipient does. This can be a challenge because it is not always easy to recognize and acknowledge emotions. Many of us, for example, have been taught that we should not feel angry. Some of us have taken that lesson so much to heart that even when our heads are pounding and our hearts are racing, even when we are sweating and shouting, we insist, "I AM NOT ANGRY!"

It can also be difficult to recognize our deeply held beliefs. Often, we take what we believe so much for granted that the way we look at the world seems to be the only way it can be viewed. Our thoughts can be so automatic that we cannot imagine a different perspective from our own. For example, we may not even realize that we hold the automatic belief that a nice person does not get angry, that we must always be nice people, and so we must never be angry. Such a set of beliefs leaves us at risk of not being able to acknowledge reasonable and natural reasons for feeling angry. Such beliefs also leave us at risk of refusing to recognize signals from our bodies or our behavior that we are angry. Not recognizing these signals or feelings can prevent us from understanding how what we are feeling motivates our behavior. However, learning to see more clearly what we feel and why can help us more effectively deal with problems that contribute to stress.

Becoming Aware of Emotions

A helpful step to becoming aware of stressful emotions is paying attention to how our bodies feel. Common signs of emotions that might be difficult to acknowledge include a pounding or racing heart, shallow or rapid breathing, headaches, sweating, tension in the neck and shoulders, clenched teeth, and stomachaches. Of course, if you are troubled by these symptoms and are concerned that they may be signs of illness—or if they cause you significant pain or interfere with your work, social or family life, or recreation—consult a healthcare professional. Even if these symptoms are related to an illness and you do get appropriate professional attention, it is helpful to examine how they may also be affected by unacknowledged emotions.

Some of our behaviors also signal that we are trying to deal with emotions of which we are unaware. For example, if we are raising our voices, scolding, sarcastically teasing others, ignoring or avoiding a person, withholding things from someone, or acting impatient, we may very well be angry.

Recognizing these signals tells us that it may be good to take different steps to deal with the things that are having such a negative impact.

The ABCs of Thinking and Feeling

The ABCs of Thinking and Feeling is a method of using what we know about emotions and thoughts to help us cope with the stress we experience when facing the challenging behaviors of others. This method assists us in looking at how our thinking can both add to our stress and help us reduce our stress. The basic idea of the ABCs of Thinking and Feeling is that when we think differently about something, we feel differently. For example, if you thought the person next to you in a crowd intentionally pushed you, you would be likely to feel differently than if you believed the person accidentally stumbled.

In the ABCs of Thinking and Feeling, "A" stands for **A**ctivating Event. This phrase reminds us that our thoughts and feelings are related to an action that happens to us or around us or that we find out about—some activating event. The previous scenario of a person pushing you is an example of an activating event.

The "B" stands for **B**eliefs, or our thoughts about the action. In the previous example, your beliefs might have been, "It was rude, mean, and obnoxious for that person to push me! That person should not do that! That person has no right to do that! It is just plain wrong!"

The "C" stands for the emotional **C**onsequences of our beliefs. Anger can be the emotional consequence of thinking that a person intentionally pushed you. Other emotional consequences include feeling stressed or upset. Even if we do not use words such as *angry*, *stressed*, or *upset*, feeling flushed or having a pounding or racing heart, or breathing rapidly, can be the emotional consequences of the action. See Handout 4.1 for a useful summary of the ABCs of Thinking and Feeling.

Anger and the ABCs of Thinking and Feeling

The challenging behaviors of those in our care can trigger feelings of anger in us. This is particularly the case when the behaviors are directed specifically toward us.

Belinda and Mr. Putin

Belinda had heard of the ABCs of Thinking and Feeling. However, when Mr. Putin yelled, "You're a G—d———— b——," what went through her mind was,

"Beliefs?! Thoughts?! I don't have any thoughts—I am just furious!" Later, at a calmer moment, she tried to use the ABCs of Thinking and Feeling to examine what happened. The "A" was easy for Belinda to identify: "Putin called me a G—d——— b——." The "C" was easy for her to identify, too: anger. Yet, it was not as easy for her to see what her thoughts were about what Mr. Putin said. "It doesn't even make sense to ask what *my* beliefs are about what *he* did," she said to herself. "It is obvious he has no right to do that. He always treats me like filth. He never acts like a human being. No matter what I do for him, he is never satisfied. I get so furious just thinking about it!"

Then Belinda realized that what she had been saying to herself were her thoughts, her beliefs. She recognized that she felt increasingly angry when she thought about what Mr. Putin had said. Her beliefs ("B") were so automatic, she had not even been considering them as thoughts. The fact that thinking about the incident increased her anger was a clue that Mr. Putin's action was not the only factor. How Belinda thought about the incident influenced how furious she felt.

A few days later, Mr. Putin called Belinda the same name while she was helping him to bed. She was startled and a little angry. Then the anger quickly passed and she felt fairly calm. She responded to Mr. Putin by saying, "You're pretty angry with me." Then she listened to him complain without trying to correct him. She knew that trying to reason with a very agitated person is not a good way of de-escalating the situation.

As Mr. Putin complained, Belinda showed she was listening, saying, "I guess I'm not very helpful sometimes," and "Oh," "Um-hmm," and, "It seems like nobody ever does what *you* want." Belinda noticed that although he continued complaining, Mr. Putin stopped shouting and cooperated as she finished helping him. In fact, he soon stopped complaining, and he said "Thank you" when Belinda was done.

Looking at what happened in this case, the "A," or the activating event, was Mr. Putin's calling Belinda a bad name. The "C," or emotional consequence, was that Belinda felt startled and a little angry, but then felt fairly calm. The emotional consequences were the result of the "B," or the beliefs or thoughts that went through Belinda's mind in reaction to Mr. Putin's strong language:

- "Who does he think he's treating this way? He should not talk to me like that!" (These were her first thoughts, which appeared to be triggered by her automatically feeling angry. These thoughts, though, seemed to intensify her anger. Then she had other thoughts as a result.)

- "Someone who acts this way has somehow learned to expect that he must be abusive to get what he wants or needs. His doing that is more likely to push people he needs away . . . or get them to retaliate."

- "He must expect that I will only pay attention if he is abusive."

- "He doesn't really know me. I make mistakes sometimes, but that doesn't make me a G—d——— b——."

- "He acts this way sometimes."

- "Yesterday we joked together while I helped him to bed. Maybe we will tomorrow, too."

Belinda's thoughts about Mr. Putin and his behavior eventually helped her avoid the stress of a very strong angry reaction. Her beliefs helped her remain fairly calm instead of feeling very angry, which in turn helped her deal with the situation effectively.

Depression and the ABCs of Thinking and Feeling

Depression is a difficult emotional experience that can be easily triggered by working with people who are in need of close care and attention. Depression is characterized by feelings of worthlessness, hopelessness, and guilt. Those suffering from depression might describe their mood as down or blue. Frequently, they have trouble with sleeping, getting too much or too little sleep. Often they have trouble eating, eating either too much or too little. People with depression often find little or no pleasure in the activities, experiences, or people they once found pleasurable. In severe cases, they can be preoccupied with thoughts of death and suicide.

Louisa and Mrs. Floyd

Louisa, a nursing assistant, was on her way to help a resident when she walked past Mrs. Floyd, who was sitting in a wheelchair in the doorway of her room. Mrs. Floyd asked if Louisa could help her to the dining room. Louisa said she would be back to help in just a few minutes. However, the other resident had a toileting mishap, so he and his clothing were quite soiled. After Louisa helped him get cleaned and changed, she rushed back toward the dining room to help residents who needed assistance eating, forgetting that she said she would help Mrs. Floyd to the dining room. While Louisa was helping another resident eat, she saw Mrs. Floyd wheel herself—slowly and with great effort—through the dining room door. Louisa then remembered her assurance of help and thought, "How horrible that I forgot. This is terrible, awful. I should not forget when I give my word that I will do something. I am undependable. I am unreliable." As she had these thoughts, she felt more and more guilty and bad about herself.

In the past, Louisa had suffered from severe depression. When she was most depressed, an incident like forgetting to go back for Mrs. Floyd would have triggered increasingly intense depressive thoughts. At those times, her thoughts were part of a downward spiral, pulling her deeper into depression. For example, she would have thoughts such as, "I should be ashamed of myself. I'm not good at my job. I don't do what I'm supposed to do. What I did to Mrs. Floyd was unforgivable." Such thinking made Louisa feel more than guilty. She would begin to feel worthless and irredeemably sinful. However, Louisa had since learned about the ABCs of Thinking and Feeling and decided to use this technique to stop her downward spiral.

The first step, being aware of how she felt, was the easiest for Louisa. It was also easy for her to know that forgetting to go back to Mrs. Floyd was the activating event that triggered her negative feelings. She had no trouble identifying the thoughts that followed the activating event, either. Louisa recorded her ABCs of Thinking and Feeling in the example that follows.

A Activating event	B Beliefs	C Emotional Consequences
I forgot to go back and help Mrs. Floyd get to the dining room.	How horrible that I forgot. This is terrible, awful. I should not forget when I give my word that I will do something. I am undependable. I am unreliable.	I felt guilty and bad about myself—a bit down.

Adding the "D" to the ABCs of Thinking and Feeling

Louisa went on to an additional step in the ABCs of Thinking and Feeling: "D." That is, she **D**isputed the thoughts that were getting her down. To do this, she questioned whether her thoughts were based on facts or just persistent beliefs. Louisa decided to look at the evidence supporting her thoughts related to the "A," or the activating event, of her forgetting to help Mrs. Floyd. She also decided to consider other ways of thinking about what happened.

"Was it really horrible, terrible, or awful that I forgot? Was anyone badly hurt? Was anything significantly damaged?" Louisa wondered. She admitted to herself that no one was physically hurt and nothing was broken. This helped Louisa recognize that she was "catastrophizing" the situation. It would be more realistic to say that she wished the incident with Mrs. Floyd had not happened rather than to consider it a catastrophe.

Louisa realized that Mrs. Floyd might have felt disappointed, angry, or down about being forgotten. She thought, "It is true that if Mrs. Floyd were forgotten like this often, it would be bad for her mental and physical health." Yet, Louisa could not recall ever having overlooked Mrs. Floyd before.

At this point in her thinking, Louisa thought, "Still, Mrs. Floyd must be very angry with me. I can't bear that. I really shouldn't do things that make anybody angry. I need people to like me." Louisa saw she was catastrophizing again, even though she was not specifically thinking the words *terrible, horrible,* or *awful.* Louisa concluded that it was not the end of the world if Mrs. Floyd got angry with her. It might be unfortunate, but it would be an understandable and survivable experience.

Louisa noticed that she was also "shoulding." Shoulding is believing that something must be, needs to be, or has to be a certain way. In this case, Louisa was shoulding by insisting that she should never do anything that upsets others. "Do I really have to not upset anyone?" she asked herself. It seemed to her that she was holding herself to an unrealistic standard. It would be more reasonable to see that not everyone will always be happy with everything she does. She has human limitations to her abilities and can therefore be expected to disappoint others at times. This is not necessarily horrible, terrible, catastrophic, or a sign that she is worthless or bad.

Louisa then considered her thought, "I need people to like me." When she thought this, she was assuming that if someone, such as Mrs. Floyd, got angry with her, that person did not like her. "If someone is angry with me for something I did, that doesn't necessarily mean that person will always be angry with me or dislike me forever," she realized. The more Louisa thought about it, the more she recognized that she was overgeneralizing. She was jumping from the idea that Mrs. Floyd would not like her to the fear that no one would. At this point Louisa thought, "Even if Mrs. Floyd doesn't like me, that doesn't mean that no one else will. It would be better if Mrs. Floyd liked me—I would really prefer that— but if she doesn't, there are other people who do."

Finally, Louisa examined the thought, "I am undependable. I am unreliable." She recognized that she was labeling herself as completely undependable and to-tally unreliable. It was true that forgetting to go back to Mrs. Floyd was not a de-pendable or reliable act. However, that did not mean that Louisa always forgot to do what she said. It did not mean she always would forget to do such tasks in the future, either. Even if Louisa did behave in undependable or unreliable ways often, she could take steps to change that.

While thinking that she was undependable or unreliable, Louisa ignored all of the times that she followed through on her word. Louisa recognized that she had been using a "mental filter," filtering out of her awareness the times when she behaved in dependable and reliable ways. She was using selective attention, noticing only what was negative. When Louisa noticed this, she made a point to recall her positive behaviors, such as helping the resident who had the toileting accident. She also did not forget to help out in the dining room. In fact, Louisa recalled many times during the day when she behaved dependably and reliably.

Disputing her initial depressing thoughts helped Louisa feel less guilty and bad about herself. She even felt less overwhelmed and tired, less stressed overall. See Handout 4.2 for a summary of the process Louisa used.

Common Unhelpful Habits of Thinking

Louisa's initial unhelpful thoughts fell into some common patterns. When we are most stressed and troubled by strong feelings such as depression, anger, or anxi-ety, we are likely to think in similar ways to Louisa. We are likely to feel most stressed when we see ourselves, others, or situations in completely negative ways. When we do this, we are thinking in either-or, all-or-nothing ways. Louisa did this when she labeled herself completely unreliable because she forgot to help Mrs. Floyd. At that time, Louisa believed she could only be either completely reliable or unreliable. There was no being partly or usually reliable; it was all or nothing. Belinda was thinking in a similar either-or, all-or-nothing way when she labeled Mr. Putin as someone who never acted like a human being. At that time, Belinda believed that a person either behaved like a human being always or never. There was no allowance for sometimes or mostly behaving like a human being.

The focus of this type of thinking affects whether we feel depressed or angry. When we focus the negative thoughts on ourselves, we are likely to feel depressed.

When our negative thoughts are focused on others, we are inclined to be angry. Any persistent or strong feelings that are harmful to our well-being, relationships, or work are likely to result from, or be contributed to by, either-or, all-or-nothing thinking.

This does not mean that emotions such as depression, anger, and anxiety can or even should be completely eliminated. They are natural, understandable feelings. It makes sense to feel angry, depressed, or anxious about some things. Eliminating such feelings may not be realistic. However, it is realistic to take steps to prevent these emotions from becoming so strong or persistent that they are hazardous to our mental or physical health, relationships, or work.

The types of unhelpful thoughts that Louisa first had illustrate some common patterns in either-or, all-or-nothing thinking. As Louisa recognized, these common unhelpful patterns of thinking included catastrophizing, shoulding, over-generalizing, using selective attention, and labeling. These thinking patterns are summarized in Handout 4.3.

Applying the ABCs of Thinking and Feeling to Your Situation

It takes practice to use the ABCs of Thinking and Feeling as well as Louisa did. Many ways of thinking that make us overly upset (unconstructively angry or depressed, for example) are habits that have developed over time. The following steps can help you learn to manage your stressful reactions to the difficult situations you face during caregiving.

Make multiple photocopies of the ABCs of Thinking and Feeling Form in the appendix to this book. Then, at the end of a day, think of one time when you were upset or stressed that day. Using one copy of the form, record how you felt (the emotional consequences) in the "C" column.

Go to column "A" and record what happened that made you upset or stressed (the activating event). Then go to the column marked "B" and record your thoughts or beliefs about the event. Ask yourself whether you were thinking in an either-or, all-or-nothing way. Were you catastrophizing, shoulding, overgeneralizing, using selective attention, or labeling?

Each day for a week, think of something that stressed or upset you that day and complete an ABCs of Thinking and Feeling Form. During the week, do not fill in the "D" column for disputing thoughts and feelings.

At the end of the week, look at each form and review your thoughts (your self-talk) about each activating event. Then question those thoughts. Keep in mind it may not be necessary to dispute all of your thoughts. For example, thoughts about how you would have preferred something to happen or thoughts about how what happened was unfortunate may be quite reasonable. These kinds of thoughts accompany periods of mild to moderate unpleasant feelings such as disappointment, regret, annoyance, or sadness. Such periodic, less-intense feelings are not problematic for health, relationships, or work. The goal of using the ABCs of Thinking and Feeling is not to eliminate all unpleasant emotional experiences. The goal is to prevent upset feelings and stress from becoming unconstructive, damaging, or harmful.

To complete the "D" section on the form—that is, to dispute the beliefs, thoughts, or self-talk listed in the "B" section—ask yourself, "What evidence supports what I think or believe about what happened?" Another helpful question is, "Are there other explanations, possibilities, or ways to think about what happened?" Again, pay particular attention to either-or, all-or-nothing thinking, and dispute catastrophizing, shoulding, overgeneralizing, using selective attention, and labeling.

Repeat this process each week, and continue using it until you notice improvement in how you usually feel or until you are better at addressing periodic difficult feelings. With this kind of practice, you may notice that you are less likely to engage in either-or, all-or-nothing thinking, and less likely to rely as heavily on unhelpful, stress-promoting ways of thinking. After a while, such formal practice may become unnecessary. If you stop practicing and notice that you are having more intense difficult feelings, begin again, using Handout 4.4 as a reference. For preliminary practice with the ABCs of Thinking and Feeling, try Exercise 4.1.

Using Our Feelings to Uncover the Motivations for Resident Behaviors

Again, the goal of using the ABCs of Thinking and Feeling is not to eliminate our feelings, but to keep our feelings from harming our overall well-being. In fact, we can use our feelings, even unpleasant ones, constructively. In our work with those who need our close care and attention, we can use our emotional reactions as clues to how best to react to their difficult behavior. Challenging behaviors have some common motivations, and caregiver reactions often mirror the feelings behind these difficult behaviors. By recognizing our feelings, we can make an educated guess about why a resident is behaving in a certain way.

The Need for Attention

We all have the need for attention, the need to feel connected to others, and the need to feel that we matter. The desire for attention is frequently related to wanting to be recognized, respected, valued, and important. A common motivation for difficult behavior is the desire for attention. When someone has a strong need for attention, he or she may call out often or have many questions or complaints that are never resolved in what the person considers a satisfactory manner. The individual may be very "chatty" as well.

Reactions to Attention-Seeking Behavior

Annoyance is a common caregiver reaction to attention-seeking behavior. A caregiver's feeling of annoyance can be a clue that the care recipient is trying to meet a need for attention. Unfortunately, it is fairly common for we as caregivers to respond out of annoyance rather than to focus on the person's need for attention.

When we respond out of annoyance, we may behave in ways that do not address the need motivating the person's behavior. We may, for example, avoid the individual. However, because he or she will likely require true assistance at some time, we will have to respond eventually. In fact, ignoring a care recipient usually reinforces his or her need for attention. Furthermore, it can also reinforce that person's belief that getting needed attention requires persistent attention-seeking behavior.

A caregiver who feels guilty about feeling annoyed may constantly respond to difficult attention-seeking behavior without a real plan to address the need in a way that will reduce the behavior. This caregiver response also tends to reinforce the difficult behavior.

Using Our Emotional Reactions to Attention-Seeking Behavior

When we use our annoyance as information about what the resident needs, we can recognize that the desire for attention is a legitimate need. The resident may be expressing it in a difficult way, but by helping him or her satisfy this need, we can reduce the difficult behaviors motivated by a desire for attention. Our plan of action can be to provide attention, especially when the resident is behaving in ways that are cooperative, helpful, and appropriately independent—or at least in ways that are not problematic. By consistently providing attention at such times, we reinforce behavior that is not difficult. In cases of attention-seeking behavior that are significant problems, we can also use the stretching method described in Chapter 3. In all cases of attention-seeking behavior, active listening can be a central part of providing the attention needed.

The Need for Power

A second common motivation for difficult behavior is the need for power. This need includes the desire to have a say in what is happening, to have an impact on others, to be able to do tasks and activities, to be able to make decisions, and to have choices. Each person has a need for power, a need to affect other people and influence the course of our lives. When a care recipient has a strong need for power, he or she may make demands rather than requests and insist that tasks be done in specific ways, at specific times, by specific people.

Reactions to Power-Seeking Behavior

Anger is a common caregiver reaction to the controlling, demanding behavior motivated by a care recipient's need for power. A caregiver's anger at the person can be a clue that the individual is trying to meet the need for power. It is fairly common, though, for caregivers to respond out of anger rather than addressing the need being expressed by the individual's behavior.

A problem with responding out of anger is that it usually does not meet the need that motivated the difficult behavior. We may, for example, persist in or increase our attempts to stay in charge. Yet this response will almost certainly reinforce the other person's need for personal power. Difficult behavior motivated by this need will then be more likely to continue or worsen as we engage in such power struggles.

Using Our Emotional Reactions to Power-Seeking Behavior

When we use our angry feelings as information, we can examine whether the person's behavior reflects the need for power. The person who depends on our care might be expressing the need in a difficult way, but effectively helping him or her satisfy the need can reduce the challenging behavior. We can help by regularly providing opportunities for care recipients to have a say in their care, including routine care, room assignments, and, in some instances, developing facility policies. Routine use of techniques described earlier for encouraging positive behavior can help caregivers address a care recipient's need for power.

The Desire for Revenge

Revenge is a third motivation for difficult behavior. We all need to receive responsive attention from others—that is, we need to see that what matters to us has an effect on those around us. When we feel that we are being neglected or made powerless, we may react by increasing attempts to get attention and exert power. If what we do does not win us attention and a sense of power, we may try to hurt those we deem responsible for the hurt we feel. We may try to make those people feel insignificant. When we are particularly vulnerable or dependent, being neglected and powerless can be very frightening. However, we often will struggle against this fear by demanding the attention and sense of power that hurting others can bring.

When a care recipient believes that attempts to get needed attention and validation of personal worth and power have persistently failed, he or she may behave in very difficult ways. For example, the person may curse and insult caregivers about their intelligence, job position, race, ethnicity, or gender. People who need care and attention, and who have severe impairments in the ability to think clearly, may even try to hit caregivers or hurt them in other physical ways. Similar violent reactions are possible from others in need of care or from people who are extremely stressed by current circumstances or life history.

Reactions to Revenge-Seeking Behavior

Caregivers often become furious in response to the hostile language or behavior of those who require close care and attention. Such a feeling can be a clue that the care recipient's ability to tolerate feeling neglected or overpowered has been severely overwhelmed. However, this clue can often be overlooked when caregivers react in anger over being attacked. For example, the staff member may angrily scold, reprimand, threaten, or insult the resident. The staff member may also increase attempts to subdue, overpower, or control the resident. The caregiver might say such things as, "I'll show you," "You won't get away with that," or "I'll give you a dose of your own medicine." When caregivers take this approach, they do not usually recognize that it is based in their own desire for revenge. A significant problem with this approach is that it frequently reinforces a resident's sense of being hurt, wronged, or mistreated. It tends to increase hostile, aggressive behavior that is motivated by the desire for revenge.

Using Our Reactions to Revenge-Seeking Behavior

Feeling furious with a care recipient can be a strong clue that the person's behavior may be motivated by the desire for revenge, and may signal that the resident feels overpowered and neglected. By tuning in to the person in our care and responding to his or her likely underlying needs, we may reduce the person's vengeful feelings and the resulting difficult behaviors. Using active listening skills and techniques for encouraging positive behavior can help the individual feel that we are paying attention and are responsive to his or her needs.

It is important to consider that in an escalating problem situation, someone may become violent. It is not permissible for a staff member to intentionally harm anyone in his or her care (for example, by using undue force to coerce compliance). It is also not permissible for a staff member to allow the individual to be harmed (by looking the other way during an escalating situation between agitated individuals, for example). A situation that involves violence by caregivers in any setting is very problematic. At the same time, it is important to take steps to avoid being physically hurt by those in your care. See Handout 4.5 for strategies on preventing physical harm by a resident.

Inadequacy

A fourth frequent motivation for challenging behavior is the feeling of inadequacy. This feeling involves a sense that it is useless to keep trying. A person who feels inadequate may believe that he or she has no worth, no effect on what is happening, and no significance to anyone. Behaviors motivated by this feeling include withdrawal, isolation, and doing little or nothing to care for oneself.

Reactions to Displays of Inadequacy

Caregivers commonly respond to an individual's displays of inadequacy by feeling hopeless and helpless in their own work with that person. They may start to see the resident as generally incapable of most or any independent tasks or activities. Caregivers may stop encouraging the person to engage in activities, including small steps in daily routines. Some caregivers may avoid the individual to avoid feeling useless.

Our responding out of feelings of futility, hopelessness, or helplessness will not address the person's underlying need for attention and need for a sense of power or competence. Not expecting or encouraging the person to do even small things can reinforce his or her feeling of inadequacy. Reducing our interaction with the individual can also make him or her feel disconnected from others. Connecting with others can go a long way in helping a person feel that needed attention is being received. Positive relationships with others can help a resident believe that he or she matters, is significant, and has an impact on others—all of which provide a sense of personal power and adequacy.

Using Our Emotional Reactions to Displays of Inadequacy

Our own feelings of futility, hopelessness, or helplessness in dealing with someone in our care can be clues that the care recipient has given up. Our goal can then be a step-by-step increase in our expectations of what he or she can do, being mindful of realistic limitations and obstacles to overcoming inadequacy while supporting effort and success along the way.

To review common motivations for difficult behavior and caregivers' common responses, see Handouts 4.6 and 4.7. Exercise 4.2 may help deepen your understanding of how to use your own reactions for clues as to what motivates others.

Breathing-Focused Relaxation

Building on the previously described stress management techniques, another helpful relaxation technique focuses simply on breathing. Like progressive muscle relaxation or mental imagery, breathing-focused relaxation can be used with other techniques or by itself. You can use it to deepen and continue your relaxation following progressive muscle relaxation or mental imagery, or it can be used alone during the 10–20 minutes you set aside each day for practicing relaxation.

First, think of a simple word or phrase, such as "calm," "peace," "one," or "I'm becoming more deeply relaxed." Pick a word or phrase that you like, one that has meaning to you and that you associate with contentment and relaxation. It will be your special word or phrase.

Sit or lie comfortably with your eyes closed. Breathe naturally, in and out. Just focus on your breathing. There is no need to make any special effort—just breathe. Each time you breathe out, say your special word or phrase. For example, breathe in and then as you exhale, say "one." Whether you say it aloud or to yourself is up to you.

As you continue to focus on breathing and repeating your word or phrase, other thoughts may enter your mind. When you notice this, return your attention to breathing and repeating your word or phrase each time you exhale. See Handout 4.8 for a quick summary of breathing-focused relaxation.

Practicing Techniques Outside of Relaxation Sessions

To get the greatest benefit from relaxation techniques, it is very helpful to practice regularly for 10–20 minutes each day. Frequently, such practice allows people to achieve deep levels of relaxation and to turn on their body's relaxation response at times other than practice sessions.

Following approximately a week of regular practice, try using your ability to relax in other situations. Keep your regular practice sessions, but add other mini sessions, using parts of the various relaxation methods at different times of the day. For example, after taking care of someone, stop to take a deep breath, inhaling as you slowly count to 5. Then exhale just as slowly and count to 10. Repeating this three times in a row can help you counteract some of the stress of your work.

Another mini session you might try is noticing where your body is most tense, such as your upper back, neck, or jaw. Wherever the muscles are most tense, let the tension go. Feel those muscles loosen and relax. You can do this at any time of the day—before working with someone who engages in challenging behavior, while walking down the hall, or during a break.

You may even focus on your breathing as it happens naturally, repeating your special word or phrase each time you exhale. You can try this for a few moments as you sit down to lunch, for instance.

It is a good idea to experiment with the different relaxation methods during the day to find how they can help you. However, remember to continue your regular daily sessions in a comfortable place where you are free from distractions. Setting aside this time may seem difficult, so give yourself credit for what you do, even if it is less than 10 minutes, and simply set a goal of gradually increasing your practice time. It is best not to get stressed out about trying to relax!

Summary

Chapter 4 covered how thinking and feeling are related to the stress of caregiving when those in our care behave in difficult ways. The chapter looked at two methods of using thoughts and feelings to manage stress. First, the ABCs of Thinking and Feeling can help us see how our thoughts about an event affect how we feel. By disputing unhelpful, stress-promoting thoughts, we can reduce our stress level. Second, realizing that our own feelings often mirror others' feelings can help us to understand what is motivating their actions. By using our emotional reactions to someone, we can make an educated guess about what is motivating the person's behavior. We can then take steps to help the individual meet the apparent need underlying the challenging behavior. This chapter also discussed breathing-focused relaxation and the importance of practicing relaxation techniques throughout the day.

The ABCs of Thinking and Feeling

It is important to cope with how we think and feel about care recipients who behave in difficult ways and about the behaviors themselves. Our thoughts or beliefs influence our emotions—that is, they influence how we feel. Often, what we feel can be described as stress. This usually means that we are having unpleasant emotions, such as anger, frustration, hopelessness, depression, anxiety, or fear. Or, it might mean we have problems, such as fatigue, muscle tension, headaches, an upset stomach, or a racing or pounding heart. (If any such symptoms are significant, speak to a healthcare professional.)

A   Our thoughts and feelings are related to an **A**ctivating Event—something that happens to us or around us or that we hear about.

A nursing home resident, Mrs. Bidwell, pulled away from Janice, a nursing assistant, and tried to hit her.

B   **B**eliefs are our thoughts about the activating event.

Janice might think, "That no-good b———! She's always trouble!" Or perhaps Janice could think, "I must not be doing what I should. I must be doing an awful job if I do it so badly that Mrs. Bidwell tries to hit me. I'm not good at anything."

C   In turn, there are emotional **C**onsequences of what we think or believe about something that happened.

If Janice thinks of Mrs. Bidwell as a "no-good b———" and a troublemaker, anger is a possible emotional consequence of what she thinks. If Janice thinks that she is doing an awful job and is not good at anything, depression could be the emotional consequence of what she thinks.

Adding the "D" to the ABCs of Thinking and Feeling

A   Our thoughts and feelings are related to **A**ctivating events—things that happen to us or around us or that we hear about.

B   Beliefs are our thoughts about the activating event.

C   In turn, there are emotional **C**onsequences of what we think or believe about something that happened.

D   We can stop and question—that is, re-evaluate and **D**ispute—the thoughts or beliefs that contribute to our stressful feelings.

Either-Or, All-or-Nothing Thinking

When we think in either-or, all-or-nothing ways, we see things, ourselves, others, or situations in extremes. For example, either-or, all-or-nothing thinking might cause us to see ourselves or someone else as always completely helpful or completely useless, rather than partly or sometimes helpful.

Common Patterns of Thinking that Can Lead to Either-Or, All-or-Nothing Thinking

Catastrophizing is seeing things as being worse than they are. Clues that we are catastrophizing include describing an event that may be unfortunate as terrible, horrible, or awful, even though limited or no harm or damage has been done as a result of the event.

Shoulding is believing that something must be, needs to be, or has to be a certain way. When we engage in this type of thinking and circumstances are not as we believe they should be, we are likely to feel very frustrated, angry, depressed, confused, or anxious.

Overgeneralizing is believing that something we have done, seen, or experienced happens much more than it actually does. We might even talk about an occasional behavior as happening all of the time.

Using Selective Attention involves seeing only certain things while ignoring others. This is like using a "mental filter," filtering some things out of our awareness. When we see only the negatives and filter out the positives, we are using selective attention.

Labeling is categorically describing things, ourselves, or others in certain ways because of some of their behaviors or characteristics. When we say that a person is bad because he or she did a bad thing, we are labeling.

Disputing Unhelpful Thoughts or Beliefs

When you are stressed or upset, notice your thoughts about whatever it is that you are stressed or upset about. Then ask, "What evidence supports what I think or believe about it? Are there other explanations, possibilities, or ways to think about it?" Answers to these questions can be used to dispute unhelpful thoughts.

Question and dispute either-or, all-or-nothing thinking. Question and dispute ways of thinking, such as catastrophizing, shoulding, overgeneralizing, using selective attention, and labeling, that can cause or contribute to an either-or, all-or-nothing point of view. The following questions are suggested for each of these types of thinking.

Catastrophizing: Is what happened really horrible, terrible, or awful? How bad was the harm or damage that was done? If there was harm or damage, can it be repaired? Would it be more accurate to say that what happened was unfortunate rather than a catastrophe?

Shoulding: Is it really true that what I am thinking is what should or must be? Won't something happen if it *must* happen? Isn't it true that expecting or demanding that reality be something other than what it is will only frustrate, anger, sadden, or disappoint me? Isn't it true that insisting that things must or should happen is holding myself and others to an unrealistic standard? Wouldn't it be more realistic to think that these are circumstances that I prefer rather than what must be?

Overgeneralizing: Is it really true that what I am upset about always happens? Does it ever *not* happen? Is it possible that if I watch carefully, I will see times when it does not happen?

Using Selective Attention: Is it really true that nothing positive happens (or that this person—or I—never do anything positive)? Is it possible that if I watch carefully, I will see positive behaviors, characteristics, or events? Is it possible that I have been overlooking positive things?

Labeling: Is it true that this person is (or that I am) completely, unchangeably _____ (fill in the blank with any unhelpful label, such as lazy, mean, incompetent, racist, sexist)? Isn't it true that people's behavior can change? Do I behave exactly the same way that I did 10 years ago? Does anyone behave in exactly the same way in all situations across his or her whole life?

Avoiding Physical Harm by a Care Recipient

1. **Be alert** to any signs that the person is getting agitated. These signs can include the individual making threats or threatening gestures, yelling, engaging in intense staring, or making repeated loud demands.

2. **Back off** when the person becomes loud or insulting, physically resists, or tries to hurt you in any situation where he or she and others are not at immediate risk of harm.

3. **Use active listening skills,** restating what you hear the person say. Allow the individual to make choices about what will happen next. It might be useful to offer limited choices such as, "Would you like me to help you now, or would it be better for me to leave?," as long as doing so does not put anyone at immediate risk of harm. Or you might say something such as, "I will be glad to help you now. But if you shout at me again, I'll know you've chosen for me to leave and come back later." With very confused and agitated people, it may be more helpful to use a calm tone of voice and describe what you are going to do as you guide and assist the person. Compliment, praise, or acknowledge positive behavior or improvements in behavior by making comments such as, "Thanks for talking to me about the problem. That helps me know what I can do to help."

4. **If the person calms down,** continue using active listening skills and other techniques for encouraging positive behavior as you provide care. If the individual does not become calm, leave him or her alone and try to provide needed care later, as long as doing so does not put anyone at risk of immediate harm.

5. **If the difficult behavior continues** when you try to offer care later, consider asking someone else, especially someone with whom the care recipient usually gets along, to stand in for you.

6. **Have two caregivers provide care in high-risk situations**. This approach is particularly useful with care recipients who are severely confused or overwhelmed. The caregivers can work as a team to distract the resident from triggers for agitation as they use active listening skills and techniques for encouraging positive behavior. Working as a team can improve care and safety when close supervision is needed for assisting very confused and easily agitated persons with activities of daily living.

7. **If a care recipient's behavior becomes an immediate, significant threat** to anyone's well-being, including your own, follow your facility's or program's policy for crisis management. When addressing such behavior in a nonprofessional care environment, have a plan in place that does not leave you alone with the individual and includes any necessary emergency telephone numbers.

Common Motivations for
the Difficult Behavior

Attention: Many difficult behaviors are motivated by the need for attention.

Power: Care recipients sometimes engage in challenging behavior when they are trying to exert power over what is happening to or around them.

Revenge: Revenge involves the desire to hurt others, or a particular person. It comes from the belief that others have, or the particular person has, hurt the individual. This a common motivation for many behaviors described as hostile, aggressive, insulting, abusive, or violent.

Feelings of inadequacy: When a care recipient feels inadequate or hopeless, he or she may not do many things effectively, including performing tasks, interacting with others, or expressing him or herself. In some cases, the person will not even try.

Source: Dinkmeyer, McKay, McKay, & Dinkmeyer (1998).

Common Caregiver Reactions to Care Recipients' Difficult Behavior

When the difficult behavior is motivated by	Caregivers often feel	And caregivers often respond by
A need for attention	Annoyed	Avoiding or withdrawing from the resident
A need for power	Angry	Insisting on being in charge
A desire for revenge	Furious	Taking the approach of "I'll show you," "You won't get away with that," or "I'll give you a dose of your own medicine." Scolding Reprimanding
A sense of inadequacy	Hopeless	Expecting the residents to do very little, if anything

These common motivations for difficult behavior are ways of being involved, of being connected and attached to others. They are ways of belonging. If a care recipient cannot establish relationships or does not know how to foster them in positive ways, he or she will likely engage in a challenging behavior.

Applying active listening skills and other techniques for encouraging positive behavior (e.g., using praise, compliments, and acknowledgment; allowing choices) instead of replying in the ways listed above can help meet care recipients' attachment needs and decrease difficult behaviors.

Source: Dinkmeyer, McKay, McKay, & Dinkmeyer (1998).

Breathing-Focused Relaxation

Practicing relaxation techniques for 10–20 minutes per day can help you manage the effects of stress. Breathing-focused relaxation can be used alone or with other relaxation methods. As with other relaxation techniques, the goal is to get as relaxed as possible without falling asleep. You can use breathing-focused relaxation to continue or deepen your relaxation by following these steps:

1. **Choose a special word or phrase,** such as "calm," "peace," "one," or "I am getting more deeply relaxed." Pick a word or phrase that you associate with contentment and relaxation.

2. **Sit or lie comfortably** in a place where you will be undisturbed for 10–20 minutes. Close your eyes and breathe naturally.

3. **Each time you exhale, say your special word or phrase.** You can say this aloud or silently—whatever works best for you.

4. **When other thoughts come into your mind,** return your focus to breathing and saying your word or phrase as you exhale.

EXERCISE 4.1

Think about an incident in which a person in your care behaved in a difficult manner about which you felt angry, depressed, or stressed. If you cannot think of such an incident involving someone in your care, think of one in which someone else behaved in a way that caused you to have a very strong negative emotional or stressed reaction. Complete the ABCD box below for the incident.

First, under "C," record how you felt about what the person did.

Next, under "A," record the difficult behavior—the activating event. Be specific. For example, rather than writing, "Mr. X refused care," it would be better to say how he did this. Perhaps, "Mr. X tried to kick me when I approached to help him out of bed."

Then, under "B," record your thoughts or beliefs about the activating event when you had your very strong negative emotional or stressed reaction. Again, be specific. For example, you might have had thoughts such as, "He can't [shouldn't, must not] do that!" "He always does things like this!" "He is just a violent person!" and "He kicks or hits everyone!"

Finally, under "D," record ideas that dispute the thoughts you listed under "B." Ask yourself questions such as, "Isn't it true that if something can't, shouldn't, or must not happen, it doesn't?" "Isn't it true that insisting that something that does happen can't, shouldn't, or must not is demanding that reality be something it is not?" "Is it true that he *always* does this?" "Aren't there any times he doesn't?" "Is it true that he is nothing but violent?" and "Isn't there anyone he doesn't kick?"

A Activating event	B Beliefs	C Emotional consequence	D Dispute beliefs

EXERCISE 4.2

Think of an incident in which a person receiving care from you behaved in a way about which you felt annoyed, angry, or helpless. If you cannot think of an incident involving a care recipient, think of one involving someone else.

Briefly describe the incident.

Briefly describe the following:

What need, desire, or feeling (e.g., the need for attention or power, the desire for revenge, or feelings of inadequacy) motivated the person's challenging behavior

What you did, or could have done, to address the need, desire, or feeling that motivated the difficult behavior

Addressing Mental Health Needs with Advance Directives and the Practice of Forgiveness

In this chapter, we will examine how advance directives provide an alternative to the use of behavior contracts in reducing or eliminating challenging behaviors. Behavior contracts are commonly used in some long-term care settings. They typically focus on rewards and imposed consequences as ways of reducing challenging behaviors. However, advance directives can also be used to proactively address the mental health, behavioral health, or stress management needs that trigger difficult behaviors. Chapter 5 also continues to develop our stress management skills. The focus will be on using forgiveness to help us with the negative feelings we can have when we are wronged. This type of stress can negatively impact how we generally feel, how we make decisions, and how we provide care. In addition to several exercises for practicing forgiveness, Chapter 5 includes another ABCs method—the ABCs of Forgiveness.

Though the first part of this chapter on using advance directives and behavior contracts is primarily intended for use in long-term care settings, it may also be helpful for nonprofessional caregivers. The second part of the chapter on using forgiveness to reduce stress is intended for all readers.

Behavior Contracts

A behavior contract in a long-term care setting is usually a written agreement between a care recipient who behaves in challenging ways and the staff or treatment team. These contracts typically say that behaving in certain positive ways will earn the resident specific privileges, such as attending therapeutic recreation activities. The contracts usually also describe which difficult behaviors will result in the loss of specific privileges. Behavior contracts are generally based on two ideas:

1. Any behaviors (including difficult behaviors) that are rewarded will increase.

2. Behaviors that have negative consequences, such as the loss of privileges, will decrease.

One significant drawback to this frequently used approach is that what some of us may describe as "rewards" are not always what trigger or reinforce a difficult behavior. In addition, negative consequences are frequently not effective at reducing or eliminating a behavior. In fact, what often appears to trigger and reinforce a difficult behavior is something the individual experiences as a negative consequence or punishment. This is so even when the staff and treatment team emphasize that their intention is not to be punitive.

The imposed consequences of behavior contracts, generally experienced as negative consequences by the care recipient, are sometimes referred to as "limit setting" by staff and consultants. Note, however, that this use of the term "limit setting" is not the same as the use of the term in this book (see Chapter 6).

Mr. Pinchbeck's case illustrates the main points discussed above.

Mr. Pinchbeck

Mr. Pinchbeck was a middle-aged long-term care resident. He was gradually losing the ability to move due to a progressive illness. Eventually he was in bed nearly all of the time. Mr. Pinchbeck needed help with toileting, bathing, dressing, and eating.

Mr. Pinchbeck had always read a great deal. He was very bright and had a very sharp, angry wit. He tried to have conversations he considered intellectual with everyone who came into his room. But then he would sarcastically insult the person, pointing out what he saw as his or her "brilliant" ignorance or stupidity. When staff members who came to his room avoided discussions with him to avoid his harsh comments, he might say something negative about the person's appearance using clearly insincere "compliments." For example, he might say something like, "I don't care what anyone says about you. You have a superior physique and they're just jealous." Or, he would say something like, "Not talking today, Einstein? I guess it's true what they say. Great minds can't do simple menial tasks and talk or chew gum at the same time."

As others increasingly stayed away from him to escape this verbal abuse, Mr. Pinchbeck would demand their attention. If they explained to him that they were avoiding him so that he could not abuse them, he would request something of them, like help with drinking some water. After sipping through his straw, he might say something like, "Thanks. Now get the f___ out of here, you pig." Staff reactions to his unpleasantness became very consistent. They withdrew from him, or ignored him, providing only the bare minimum of required care. Mr. Pinchbeck's hostile comments and insults became his usual way of dealing with anyone who came into his room.

After some months of very little interaction with anyone, beyond receiving very quick and silently given daily care, Mr. Pinchbeck expressed an interest in something he had been reluctant to try earlier. He requested a motorized wheelchair, one specifically customized to his abilities. In response to his request, the treatment team decided to offer Mr. Pinchbeck a behavior contract. The members of the team met with Mr. Pinchbeck at his bedside to explain the contract to him. They described how he would need to complete training for using a chair safely before he could get his own wheelchair. He would need to have "driving lessons" before a chair was ordered specifically for him. Once he demonstrated his ability to use a wheelchair safely, one would be ordered for him.

Then the team explained how the behavior contract would be part of Mr. Pinchbeck getting the wheelchair. He was told that prior to each step along the way to getting and using the chair, he would have to use respectful language with staff and refrain from using harsh language and insults for at least 2 weeks. For example, for 2 weeks prior to his first lesson in using a motorized wheelchair, Mr. Pinchbeck would need to speak respectfully to staff and avoid any offensive, hostile, or insulting language.

As the treatment team explained these conditions of the behavior contract, Mr. Pinchbeck became enraged. Using a torrent of the strongest obscenities and referring to the staff as tyrants and petty dictators, he demanded that they all leave his room. For months after this interaction, the intensity and frequency of Mr. Pinchbeck's difficult behavior increased significantly.

In Mr. Pinchbeck's case, the treatment team intended to use wheelchair practice sessions as rewards for positive behavior. They planned to withhold these sessions so as not to reward Mr. Pinchbeck's difficult behavior of using hostile, insulting language. They described their approach as "limit setting." However, his difficult behavior increased when what he had requested was withheld. Mr. Pinchbeck explained that this was his way of defying what he experienced as the team's tyranny and dictatorship. Mr. Pinchbeck saw the team's behavior contract as an attempt by others to control him, which to him was a punishment.

Observing Mr. Pinchbeck's behavior using the ABCs of Behavior and active listening indicated that there was a common theme in the events that triggered and reinforced his difficult behavior. They were typically situations that heightened his awareness of his disability, his powerlessness, and his sense of not being who he believed he was supposed to be—a capable, strong person.

A more accurate assessment of the triggers and reinforcers of Mr. Pinchbeck's challenging behavior would have shown that the use of a behavior contract, as such contracts are widely used, was likely to result in the opposite of the treatment team's expressed intention.

This approach to behavior contracts is likely to be just as unhelpful in other cases for several reasons. First, such contracts are not useful in cases where the care recipient is unable to understand the details of the contract. Second, they are not helpful when the person does not see his or her difficult behavior as a problem, but as a right, justified, or appropriate response. Third, behavior contracts are similarly not effective in cases where the person denies that the difficult behaviors even happen. Fourth, behavior contracts often have results opposite to what would be good outcomes when the person with challenging behaviors sees the contract as an attempt to control him or her. The circumstances indicated that this was the case with Mr. Pinchbeck.

When behavior contracts are part of an ongoing power struggle, it is unlikely they will lead to positive behavior. In such instances, they are more likely to reinforce agitated challenging behavior or behavior that shows helplessness. They may also lead to a type of compliance on the part of the care recipient that is sometimes described by staff as "pretending" or "manipulative." Such outcomes do not promote the well-being of the resident. They also do not promote a positive, therapeutic long-term care culture.

When behavior contracts are followed by persistent or increasingly agitated or hostile behavior, this can lead to greater efforts by staff to control the resident. Common ways of doing this include the use of such restraining methods as medication, restriction to bed, or admission to locked units. These methods are often endorsed by overly stressed staff, administrators, and consultants who are trying to use behavior contracts to guide the treatment of a resident's difficult behavior. At such times, a statement often made is "nothing else works."

Behavior contracts may be helpful to some degree when they are made with someone who agrees that the behaviors others see as difficult are indeed problems. In addition, the person would want to change those behaviors and be in full, free support of the contract. Such contracts will also only be effective if they are based on an accurate assessment of the triggers and reinforcers of the difficult behavior. Such an assessment should include using techniques such as the ABCs of Behavior and active listening.

The following section outlines an alternative approach to using behavior contracts to address the issue of challenging behaviors in long-term care. This approach is designed to avoid the many limitations of the typical behavior contract.

Advance Directives

An alternative to the commonly used behavior contract is another type of agreement between a long-term care setting, care staff, and a resident. This alternative type of agreement is called an advance directive.

Advance directives are written instructions that care recipients give to those who provide care to them. These instructions include information such as what types of healthcare treatment a person does and does not want. Advance directives are created when the individual is able to think clearly enough to make informed decisions. These instructions are used later when the person is unable to make informed decisions or is unable to communicate what treatment he or she does or does not want.

Many healthcare settings in the United States, such as hospitals and long-term care communities, are required by law to have policies and procedures in place that help care recipients document their advance directives. In addition, in many places it is legally required that these directives be followed unless what the individual wants is clearly inappropriate healthcare. A healthcare professional who has a moral objection to following a specific advance directive may, typically, refuse to carry it out. However, when a healthcare professional has a moral objection to following the individual's wishes, then he or she may have a legal obligation to transfer the care of the person to a healthcare professional who is able to follow the individual's wishes according to the American Bar Association (American Bar Association Commission on Law and Aging, http://www.americanbar.org).

Although advance directives are typically used to guide end-of-life decisions, they can and increasingly do guide the care people receive for mental health issues. Mental health issues are common in long-term settings and are frequently related to the challenging behaviors of care recipients. Using advance directives to address the mental health needs of care recipients can be an important approach to reducing or eliminating challenging behaviors.

Mental Health Advance Directives

Mental health advance directives are agreements between care recipients and healthcare providers. These providers include physicians, nurses, nursing assistants, and the entire staff of a healthcare or long-term care setting or program. Mental health advance directives typically have the same legal standing as general healthcare advance directives.

There is an important issue in some places where mental health advance directives policies and procedures are legally required. In these jurisdictions, employees in care settings cannot legally assist care recipients to document mental health advance directives. The same is true of close family members in some jurisdictions. These places require that a third party provide that assistance.

It is important that the administrative leaders in a long-term care facility or program get legal counsel to ensure that the laws in their areas are followed. This can enable those leaders to ensure that staff members are given the necessary guidance, information, and education about how mental health advance directives are obtained. Before following the approach to documenting advance directives described in this book, check the legal requirements for your setting.

As with healthcare advance directives in general, a person makes mental health advance directives at a time when he or she is able to think clearly enough to make informed healthcare decisions and is able to communicate them. With mental health advance directives, care recipients provide instructions about what types of treatment they do and do not want to receive for mental health issues that might arise. Like general advance directives, mental health advance directives also allow the person to identify someone else to make care decisions for him or her if, at any time, he or she cannot make or express informed decisions. Advance directives are intended to take effect whenever the individual cannot clearly communicate his or her wishes to others.

There are cases where a person has not made advance directives by the time he or she might need them. It is not uncommon in such cases that the person has also not indicated who he or she would like to make decisions when he or she is not able to think clearly enough or cannot communicate decisions. Typically there are legal guidelines for deciding who will be able to make treatment decisions for the individual in such cases. These guidelines usually indicate that the next of kin or a legally appointed guardian or advocate will make treatment decisions. Here, again, it is important that the administrative leaders of facilities or programs get legal counsel to be sure that the practices in their settings are in line with the laws in their locations.

Indications of Mental Health Needs

There are several indications that a care recipient has, or is at increased risk of having, unmet mental health needs and that advance planning is called for. A diagnosed severe mental illness is one obvious indication, however, it is not the only indication. There are at least three other broad categories of indications that the person's mental health needs are currently unmet in long-term care settings and programs:

- If a person has persistent troubling emotions that undermine a generally positive experience of life, this is a mental health issue, even if a mental illness has not been diagnosed.

- Limited involvement in activities that give a person a sense of having a meaningful life is also an indication that attention to the individual's mental health is needed.

- Difficulty getting along with others is another important indication that a person's mental health needs attention.

The challenging behaviors of those receiving long-term care are often related to one or more of these three categories of mental health issues. Since these issues are widespread in long-term care settings or programs, it is critical that steps to address them become a routine duty of all those working in long-term care.

One way to proactively address the mental health needs of a resident is to incorporate into the process of documenting advance directives a discussion of how he or she would like these issues addressed. The following example illustrates how a resident introduced in Chapter 1 could have been assisted in making mental health advance directives, had such advance directives been used.

Mr. D'Angelo and Chaplin Dworkin

Mr. D'Angelo was losing his ability to remember things and to think clearly. He had a diagnosis of probable Alzheimer's disease. Although Mr. D'Angelo was having more difficulty remembering things and difficulty thinking clearly at the time he was admitted to the long-term care residence, he was still able to remember and think clearly enough to make informed decisions about his healthcare, including his mental healthcare.

For several years, Chaplain Dworkin had been a part of the long-term care residence to which Mr. D'Angelo was admitted. The chaplain was valued and re-spected widely among the staff. Chaplain Dworkin had training and experience in discussing end-of-life advance directives with residents. He was often the person who helped them document those directives. Recently, Chaplain Dworkin had sought out and received training in helping residents to complete mental health advance directives.

The Chaplain knew that Mr. D'Angelo had not wanted to complete any advance directives prior to being admitted. When Chaplain Dworkin visited with Mr. D'Angelo, he took time to chat and get to know him. Eventually their conver-sation included talking about what kind of medical care Mr. D'Angelo would and would not want if, for example, he was found not breathing and without a pulse. Mr. D'Angelo let the chaplain know that he really did want his wishes to be fol-lowed in those situations. The chaplain's positive relationship with Mr. D'Angelo helped Mr. D'Angelo to think through and express his wishes. Chaplain Dworkin visited with Mr. D'Angelo a few times and helped him document his wishes for end-of-life treatment.

The chaplain continued to visit with Mr. D'Angelo, furthering the positive relationship with him. Mr. D'Angelo responded very well to Chaplain Dworkin's active-listening style of interacting. During these visits, Mr. D'Angelo spoke of his interactions with others and how his increasing reliance on others affected his self-esteem, making him feel down or angry. Mr. D'Angelo admitted that he sometimes was not very easy to get along with because he was having difficulty with his feelings about his current life circumstances.

Mr. D'Angelo also described how he was thinking less and less clearly, be-coming more easily confused, and having increasing difficulty with his memory. He said he felt like he was losing himself, which made him feel very sad and scared. At times, he would start to feel so overwhelmed by these feelings that he would fight to avoid them; whenever someone seemed to be on the side of "the deterioration process," interfering with his sense of being a capable, worthwhile person, he would behave irritably and uncooperatively as a way to fight against what was happening to him. His fear would trigger this rebellious behavior since he saw no other way of preventing what he described as his "decline." He would become so focused on a perceived threat that he would not listen to reason.

During the conversation, Chaplain Dworkin restated some of the feelings and beliefs that Mr. D'Angelo was describing: "It's important to you to have a say in what is happening to or even around you. It's important that you have choices. When others really listen and really understand you, their understanding has a very positive effect on how you feel and on the things you do. You feel respected when the people you depend on show that they recognize and appreciate positive things you do. When people understand that how you feel, what you think, and how you behave is affected by your interactions with them, you feel deeply connected to them, and that can feel good."

Chaplain Dworkin said, "Positive relationships are good for your mental health." He went on to explain that this is true for everyone. The more stress we experience, the more important positive relationships are for helping us decrease unpleasant feelings of depression, anxiety, or anger. "They are good medicine," Chaplain Dworkin said. He added that positive relationships are central to good healthcare.

The chaplain explained that it is important for caregivers in a long-term care community to know how to help improve a resident's mental health. He described how it can also be very helpful for a resident to make clear to staff what he does and does not want done in order to help him with feeling down, nervous, or irritable and with any unpleasant, stressful feelings. It is sometimes easier and other times harder for a resident to let a caregiver clearly know that something the caregiver is doing is having either a positive or negative effect. The chaplain also said that there are times when a resident is so stressed, confused, or ill that the person cannot communicate how he or she wants to be treated to address problems in how he or she is feeling, thinking, or behaving. There are also times when a resident is thinking clearly, but still cannot communicate his or her wishes. At these times, it is helpful to have these wishes written down.

At this point, Chaplain Dworkin offered to help Mr. D'Angelo write down his mental health advance directives. Mr. D'Angelo said that he was uncomfortable with calling his needs "mental health" needs. He agreed with the chaplain that it was valid to call the needs they had been discussing "stress management needs" instead. Chaplain Dworkin said he could help Mr. D'Angelo document his stress management instructions for staff about how he would want to be treated to deal with stress, strong troubling emotions (for example, depression, anxiety, or anger), and any challenging behaviors motivated by such distress. These instructions would be intended for use any time Mr. D'Angelo was unable to communicate his wishes clearly or was unable to think clearly enough to make decisions about his care.

Mr. D'Angelo said he was very interested in doing that. The chaplain continued by pulling out a form that would help document advance directives in terms that would be most comfortable for the care recipient. Chaplain Dworkin explained to Mr. D'Angelo that they could use the form to document Mr. D'Angelo's wishes. Based on his discussions with Mr. D'Angelo, Chaplain Dworkin believed he already knew how Mr. D'Angelo would respond to many of the questions on the form. "But just to make sure, I'll go over each of the questions with you," the chaplain said.

To see a section from the form Chaplain Dworkin would have used in this hypothetical scenario, refer to Handout 5.1, which details Part 1A of the Advance Directives: MH/BH/SM Form (Advance Directives: Mental Health/ Behavioral Health/Stress Management Form). In addition to the Part 1A section shown, some other sections of the form will be introduced in handouts later in this chapter. The entire form is available in the appendix of this book.

The case of Ms. Oakley that follows is an example of how a next of kin or healthcare proxy could provide the type of information required by mental health advance directives in cases where the care recipient never completed such advance directives before they were needed.

Ms. Oakley

Ms. Oakley was introduced in Chapter 3. Age 75, she typically stayed in her room, talking with someone no one else could see. Ms. Oakley had a diagnosis of schizophrenia from the time she was young. When Ms. Oakley spoke, it was generally very difficult to understand what she said. She usually mumbled when she did say recognizable words, and the words were not typically put into sentences that made sense to others.

In Chapter 3, we learned that Ms. Oakley's long-term care community was temporarily understaffed. Ms. Oakley was discovered to have had a toileting mishap. Sitting in her soiled clothing on the floor, she was wiping feces from her hands onto her bedspread. Miki, a licensed practical nurse, rushed in and loudly directed Ms. Oakley to stop what she was doing. Miki grabbed Ms. Oakley's arm. Startled, Ms. Oakley hit Miki. Because of this incident, Ms. Oakley's antipsychotic medication was increased.

Although mental health advance directives were not used in Ms. Oakley's case, the incident with Miki could have been an opportunity to document her needs for any future incidents. Since being admitted to the facility, Ms. Oakley had not shown she was able to understand healthcare information, including mental healthcare options. However, her sister and next of kin, Ms. Kim, could. Ms. Kim was legally permitted to make healthcare decisions for Ms. Oakley. The following scenario describes how a discussion between Ms. Kim and the nurse manager, Joan, could have been used to document mental health advance directives for Ms. Oakley.

Ms. Kim, Ms. Oakley's Sister

Ms. Kim visited her sister, Ms. Oakley, regularly. At the long-term care community, Ms. Kim routinely attended care planning team meetings about her sister. Although these meetings were always very busy and there was little time for discussion, Ms. Kim politely asked questions to better understand her sister's care. She also asked what she could do to help with her sister's care. After the incident between Ms. Oakley and Miki, Ms. Kim was asked to meet with Joan, the new nurse manager, to discuss what had happened. Joan hoped to hear Ms. Kim's ideas about the best ways to approach any future episodes of difficult behavior from Ms. Oakley.

In her meeting with Ms. Kim, Joan explained what happened. Ms. Kim replied that she was very sorry that her sister had behaved in such an alarming way and asked if the staff member had been hurt.

"No," Joan said, "but the staff member was shaken up a bit."

"Anyone would be," Ms. Kim responded. "I really am sorry this happened."

Joan told Ms. Kim that although she had just started working at the long-term care community, she had learned that there had been a couple of similar incidents when Ms. Oakley was first admitted about 2 years earlier. Joan explained that she knew this from looking back in Ms. Oakley's chart and talking with staff members who had been at the facility for several years.

Ms. Kim knew about these earlier incidents and had been asked to meet with the nurse manager then, too. Ms. Kim described how she and the previous nurse manager discussed the incidents and what Ms. Kim thought might be the best approach to reducing or eliminating Ms. Oakley's challenging behaviors. As she and Joan talked, Ms. Kim expressed that she appreciated the way the previous nurse manager and Joan had asked for her input.

Ms. Kim explained that Ms. Oakley had spent much of her life in hospitals because of her schizophrenia. "There were many very caring people in those places," she said. "But the resources were always very limited and there was very little guidance for the people who were in the most direct contact with patients like my sister. My sister did not really get the best care in those hospitals." Ms. Kim described how staff in those settings said Ms. Oakley was "really hard to handle."

However, Ms. Kim also said that in the few years before Ms. Oakley's admission to the long-term care community, when she was in a group home, she rarely engaged in problematic behaviors. "It was very different from the hospitals she'd been in up to that time," Ms. Kim said. Ms. Oakley's difficult behaviors were minor and infrequent in the group home. "In fact," Ms. Kim said, "my sister was on less medication during her stay in the group home than she'd been on in a very long time."

Ms. Kim said that during her visits to the group home to see her sister she learned a great deal by watching the staff there. Although Ms. Oakley generally kept to herself, the staff checked in with her regularly and frequently. A staff member checking in with Ms. Oakley would take a couple of minutes just to sit with Ms. Oakley. Ms. Oakley was also encouraged to do simple chores, such as putting laundry away, which she was usually able to do for a few minutes with guidance and positive encouragement before quietly walking away.

"My sister didn't get to the point of doing much by herself, but her behavior was so much better than it had been, and she really was able to be with people more than she'd been in years," Ms. Kim said.

"So when she wasn't left alone for long periods and staff members interacted with her as much as she was able to tolerate, your sister made what might've seemed like small gains to an outside observer who did not know her. You could see, though, how important those changes were," Joan said.

"Yes, that's right," Ms. Kim responded, "and the times when she was fussy were usually when her routine was changed, like when a staff member who had worked closely with her got a new job and left the group home."

Joan asked, "Can you tell me more about what you mean when you say, 'fussy'?"

"Well, one time I was visiting my sister shortly after our mother had died. A new staff member had taken over for Betsy, who had been caring for my sister for some time, but had recently switched jobs. My sister was in her pajamas and standing silently looking at the wall. The new person said, 'Okay, Ms. O., it's time to get washed and dressed.' My sister didn't respond. The staff member said she'd check back in a little while. I got some of her clothes from the closet and said these might be nice to wear that day, but my sister didn't react to me.

"When the staff member came back, my sister had still not washed and dressed, even though she was capable of doing these tasks herself. The staff member said, 'Why don't we pick out what you'd like to wear today.' Still, my sister did not respond. She did not move and did not look at the staff member or me. The staff member then said, 'Okay, dear, maybe we can find something nice in the closet,' and took my sister's hand. My sister quickly jerked her hand away and stepped closer to the wall she was facing."

Joan asked how the situation was resolved. Ms. Kim explained that the staff member said she could see that Ms. Oakley did not want to get dressed just then, that she seemed to want to be alone. The staff member added, 'I guess it's hard when someone you've known for a long time, someone who matters to you, is gone. It can be very difficult to get to know someone new, like me.' Then the staff member left.

Ms. Kim went on to explain that about an hour after the staff member left the room, she returned with another person, Jill, who had worked at the group home for some time. Jill had been friendly with Betsy, the staff member who left for a new job. Jill and Betsy had worked very well together with Ms. Oakley.

Jill said to Ms. Oakley, "I miss Betsy, too. I feel sad and angry that she's gone." Jill asked Ms. Oakley if she wanted to pick out some clothes for the day or whether she would prefer that Jill pick them out. When Ms. Oakley did not respond, Jill said, "Okay, let's see, how about this. You don't have to pick out your clothes. If you don't pick, that can be the way you let me know that you'd like me to pick them out." Then Jill held up two shirts and asked which one Ms. Oakley would like to wear. Ms. Oakley pointed to the dark blue one, which was her favorite color.

Using active listening, Joan restated what she thought Ms. Kim was saying. She said, "So the staff's actions helped ensure that your sister's difficult behavior—which might have been described as noncompliance or agitatedly resisting care—did not escalate. The new staff member showed she was listening to your sister by considering recent changes and what was happening in the moment when she said, 'I guess it's hard when someone who is important to you is gone,' and, 'It can be difficult to get to know someone new.' She also showed she had been listening when she went and got someone else who was familiar to your sister. That person, Jill, interacted with your sister in ways that demonstrated she thought she understood what Ms. Oakley was dealing with—missing Betsy. I suspect that Jill also kept in mind that your mother had recently died. Jill also respected your sister's right to make decisions. She saw that your sister was stressed and seemed unable to select her outfit when her options were too broad. She helped your sister by offering her guidance on getting dressed, but also by providing Ms. Oakley a limited choice that was within her ability to make.

"It appeared that these approaches of empathically listening and of encouraging positive behavior by framing choices according to your sister's ability and behaviors were very effective."

Mental Health Advance Directives in Ms. Oakley's Case

Ms. Kim gave Joan a good deal of insight into Ms. Oakley. This information, along with Ms. Oakley's history at the long-term care residence, helped Joan supervise staff members who worked with Ms. Oakley. Joan's job may have been easier if mental health advance directives for Ms. Oakley had been documented at the time of her admission, or shortly after.

Although Ms. Oakley had never demonstrated that she was able to understand information and make informed healthcare decisions while at the long-term care residence, her sister, Ms. Kim, clearly did. As an involved and caring next of kin, Ms. Kim would have been the appropriate person to create advance directives to guide Ms. Oakley's mental healthcare. Her input would have highlighted that Ms. Oakley's difficult behavior was likely to be triggered not only by her schizophrenia, but also by external events.

The mental health advance directive that Ms. Kim, or another designated healthcare proxy, might have documented would have had the same legal and ethical standing as any mental health advance directives created by Ms. Oakley. In such a case, the Advance Directives: MH/BH/SM Form could be used. To complete the form, the next of kin or the designated healthcare proxy would fill in Part 1B and other relevant sections to indicate treatment preferences. Handout 5.2 shows Part 1B of the Advance Directives: MH/BH/SM Form, which appears in the appendix.

The next case is another example of how a direct discussion early on of mental health/behavioral health/stress management advance directives may generally help with addressing a care recipient's mental health needs.

Mrs. Lowenthal

In Chapter 2, we learned about the case of Mrs. Lowenthal. She was 100 years old, nearly completely blind, and had diminishing hearing. Mrs. Lowenthal was so frail that she could not stand or walk on her own. For some time following her arrival at the long-term care community, Mrs. Lowenthal stayed in her room alone, turning down invitations to join in therapeutic recreation and to have her meals in the dining room. Mrs. Lowenthal acknowledged that she was very depressed. Several months after her arrival, a licensed practical nurse, Teresa, was assigned to deliver medications to the residents on Mrs. Lowenthal's hall. This was the first time Teresa worked with Mrs. Lowenthal.

Teresa connected with Mrs. Lowenthal by skillfully using active listening and developing a deep empathic understanding of Mrs. Lowenthal, her life, and her emotions. Teresa's approach encouraged Mrs. Lowenthal to be more engaged, first with Teresa, then with other staff. Later, Mrs. Lowenthal developed friendships with three other residents. Clearly, there was an improvement in Mrs. Lowenthal's depression.

It is a common misperception that the only ways of treating mental health issues, including depression, are psychotherapy or medication. Both psychotherapy and medication can be very helpful treatment options in many instances in long-term care settings. In most cases, however, they should typically be considered adjuncts to a proactive and responsive long-term care environment made up of people such as Teresa, whose interactions with residents are routinely therapeutic. The staff are the central component of a therapeutic environment in a well-functioning long-term care setting.

Mrs. Lowenthal's long-term care community did not use mental health advance directives, so Mrs. Lowenthal did not have her wishes documented in this way. However, she did clearly and repeatedly say that she did not want medication for her depression and did not want to talk with any mental health professional. Mrs. Lowenthal had also said, less directly, that she would prefer to have staff engage in genuine listening, listening that would help them to deeply and empathically connect with her in ways that would decrease her sense of isolation, helplessness, and worthlessness. It took a number of months before Mrs. Lowenthal's indirect manner of expressing her wishes was understood and responded to thanks to Teresa.

If Mrs. Lowenthal had had the opportunity to create her mental health advance directives at the time of, or shortly after, her admission, it is possible that staff would have effectively responded to her depression earlier. Although mental health advance directives are generally intended to provide instructions for times when a person is unable to make healthcare decisions or is unable to communicate them, these advance directives can also provide general guidance in understanding a care recipient's typical preferences—preferences that can inform how to *routinely* provide for the individual's mental healthcare.

Handout 5.3 features the Essentials of Care section of the Advance Directives: MH/BH/SM Form. This section provides an opportunity for long-term care staff, treatment teams, and care recipients to collaboratively establish a process for routinely and proactively addressing mental health, behavioral health, and stress management needs in long-term care.

The Essentials of Care section would have been appropriate to use not only in Mrs. Lowenthal's case, but also in each of the previously discussed cases of Mr. D'Angelo, Ms. Oakley, and Mr. Pinchbeck. The additional case that follows of Ms. Quigley emphasizes the value of using mental health advance directives that include the Essentials of Care as a central component for each care recipient.

Ms. Quigley

Ms. Quigley was another long-term care resident who is described in Chapter 1. Ms. Quigley was 77 years old and had increasing difficulty breathing. This difficulty was caused by chronic obstructive pulmonary disease. Her illness progressed for a number of years before she was admitted to the long-term care residence. Ms. Quigley was generally quite anxious and fearful because of the difficulty she had breathing. The more fearful she felt, the more she called out for attention. Even when her breathing was relatively stable, it was still impaired and continued to make her anxious. She often called for staff to help her, even with tasks that she was able to do on her own. Staff members found it difficult to respond to Ms. Quigley's frequent requests for attention.

For many weeks, the staff followed a plan devised to reduce Ms. Quigley's calling out for attention. The plan was to avoid responding to Ms. Quigley's calls when there was no immediate need regarding her health, her safety, or her routine activities of daily living, such as toileting, bathing, dressing, and eating. However, this plan did not include attending to Ms. Quigley's routine mental health needs, as described in this book. Instead, this plan was based simply on the idea that responding to her calls was rewarding her frequent calls for attention.

Unfortunately, the plan did not reduce the intensity or frequency of Ms. Quigley's attention-seeking behavior. Instead, there was an increase in panic attacks (episodes of severe anxiety), which included marked impairment in breathing. Because there were a number of factors reinforcing Ms. Quigley's attention-seeking behavior, focusing on just one possible reinforcer, responding to her calls, was unlikely to reduce the behavior.

Ms. Quigley's calls for attention appeared significantly related to her fear, but not just to the staff response she received when she called. Her fear was triggered and reinforced by her impaired breathing. Her beliefs about her declining ability to breathe and how her illness would progress until she died also seemed to contribute to her difficult behavior: "I know that no one can help me stop that, stop my breathing from getting worse. Being hooked up to oxygen when I've needed it always helped at first, but even at the maximum setting now, I don't get much relief. Some of my medications had made it easier to breathe, but they don't work as well as they used to. The ones that were the most helpful had the side effect of making me even more anxious. Some of the pills to calm me down helped, but now they make it even harder to breathe."

Ms. Quigley said the one thing that reduced her fear and anxiety was being with someone who was not upset or overwhelmed by how she was feeling and behaving, but instead understood and cared about her. Ms. Quigley knew that her anxiety and fear made it difficult for others to be around her, but being alone only made her feel more frightened and more inclined to call out for help.

Ms. Quigley explained all this to Peggy, a social worker. After many weeks of following the staff's original plan for reducing Ms. Quigley's calls for attention, the plan was revised based on what Ms. Quigley had said to Peggy. The new, revised plan reflected Peggy's and Ms. Quigley's use of cooperative problem solving. Peggy's role in the new plan was to encourage Ms. Quigley to express herself and to allow Ms. Quigley choices whenever they were together.

Eventually the treatment plan for Ms. Quigley's difficult behavior included, in addition to Peggy's regular 15-minute visits twice a week, frequent brief visits to

Ms. Quigley from staff members assigned to care for her daily. Each staff member made at least one visit a day that was at least 2–3 minutes long. The focus of these visits was not on routine care tasks such as activities of daily living, administering medications, or checking vital signs. All of these necessary tasks were done during other visits. Instead, staff members, important people in Ms. Quigley's life, would spend these consistent, short visits using active listening skills and responding to Ms. Quigley with empathy. With this new treatment plan, staff *routinely* addressed Ms. Quigley's mental health needs in the same way they would address routine activities of daily living. Staff also acknowledged that by attending to common, expected problems that residents experience related to living among other long-term care residents is an important part of addressing another routine activity of daily living—stress management.

Eventually, Ms. Quigley was receiving brief daily visits from her nursing assistants, licensed practical nurses, charge nurses, nurse practitioners, housekeepers, recreation therapists, occupational therapy assistants, food service workers, and Peggy. Ms. Quigley was still never completely free from her anxiety or fear. However, she had fewer panic attacks and called out less often for much of her time at the long-term care residence. There were times when the frequency of her panic attacks and episodes of calling out increased, but only when there was a notable decline in her ability to breathe.

The original treatment plan for addressing Ms. Quigley's difficult behavior was revised based on Peggy's visits with Ms. Quigley months after she arrived at the long-term care residence. It is possible that a similarly effective plan would have been made earlier if Ms. Quigley had been helped to document mental health advance directives, at or shortly after her admission. As with each of the cases discussed earlier, the Essentials of Care section in the Advance Directives: MH/BH/SM Form (Handout 5.3) could have been used as a guide for documenting Ms. Quigley's preferences.

In the earlier case with Mr. D'Angelo, he received help with completing his mental health advance directives from a chaplain. This support role of helping develop mental health advance directives can sometimes be filled by someone such as Peggy, the social worker in Ms. Quigley's case. However, as mentioned previously, please note that in some settings where mental health advance directives are legally required, employees of those settings are prohibited from assisting with the documentation of mental health advance directives. In these settings, a third party must provide assistance to the care recipient in documenting mental health advance directives. Be sure to check the legal requirements for your setting.

Grievances and Stress

Later in this chapter, we will discuss how practicing forgiveness can relieve grievance-related stress. First, we will review how grievances are linked to stress and how a grievance-based perspective can negatively influence treatment plans and the use of behavior contracts.

It is very common for us to experience grievance-related stress after someone treats us unfairly or insults or harms us in some way. When someone has wronged us, we may feel irritated, angry, outraged, hurt, hopeless, unhappy, depressed, anxious, or frightened or a combination of all of these unpleasant emotions. This would be a grievance reaction, that is, a largely emotional reaction to the way we were treated.

There is a range of common reactions to being treated harshly, rudely, unkindly, or poorly. Many of us are usually well aware of how we feel about being wrongly treated, and we recognize when these strong and persistent feelings are causing us stress. However, for some of us, when we are wronged we are not fully aware of the specific emotions underlying our stress. In these cases, we may feel a vague stress, a sense of discomfort, tension, or fatigue. We may feel irritable, down, or anxious, but not be aware of the link between those feelings and how we have been treated.

At other times, some of us may not even be aware of our stress. If we pay close attention to our feelings, thoughts, and actions, we may notice that we are experiencing unacknowledged stress. One major sign of unacknowledged stress is behavior that negatively impacts others or ourselves. Such behavior may include withdrawing from others, becoming overly focused on completing concrete tasks, ignoring others, and insisting, demanding, or arguing. This behavior may be accompanied by a sense of indifference, numbness, or "objective" detachment.

We may experience any of the above reactions to being wronged, all of which can lead to a sense of stress. See Handout 5.4 for a summary of the common indications that we are experiencing grievance-related stress. Use Exercise 5.1 to practice recognizing common reactions to being wrongly treated.

Grievances can also negatively influence treatment decisions and formal treatment plans. Approaches to challenging behaviors that are significantly influenced by a grievance-based perspective are typically ineffective and are often even triggers and reinforcers of the behavior. A plan or behavior contract that is affected by staff grievances can lead to an approach focused on holding the care recipient "accountable" for his or her challenging behaviors (that is, having the individual experience a negative cost), rather than working toward the goal of simply reducing or eliminating the behaviors. The following case of Mr. Callahan details how a grievance-based perspective to behavior contracts and treatment plans can negatively impact care and even increase challenging behaviors.

Mr. Callahan

Mr. Callahan was introduced in Chapter 2. Although he had suffered a stroke, his initial recovery went well. Early in his recovery, he regained enough use of his left leg to stand with assistance. Later, with help, he was able to walk up and down a hallway with an uneven gait. However, he never regained the ability to raise his left arm without assistance or grasp with his left hand.

Mr. Callahan often complained that he was not treated well or fairly. He frequently insulted staff members and other residents. Mr. Callahan's wife and adult children said that such behavior was typical of him. They described how Mr. Callahan had always been critical, demanding, and dissatisfied with what others did for him. However, his family also explained that Mr. Callahan hated being alone, even though he typically argued or insulted others when he was with them.

In Chapter 2, we saw how staff members responded effectively in one instance to reduce the intensity of Mr. Callahan's challenging behavior. In that example, Don, a nursing assistant, used active listening. He rephrased what he thought Mr. Callahan was expressing through his words and behavior while ignoring the difficult behavior. Don was able to "hold on" and not act on the anger he understandably felt—anger that appeared to mirror Mr. Callahan's own feelings.

Don felt angry because he felt attacked by Mr. Callahan. Reflecting on his own emotional response, Don realized that Mr. Callahan probably also experienced the situation as an attack on him. Don guessed that responding in a demanding, insisting, controlling, or counter-aggressive way would only reinforce Mr. Callahan's perception that he was being attacked and lead to an escalation of the troubling situation. Don not only listened to how Mr. Callahan felt, he also listened for what triggered Mr. Callahan's anger.

Before Don had been assigned to work with Mr. Callahan, there were a number of incidents in which Mr. Callahan's angry, demanding, insulting behavior escalated to his screaming threats. In one instance, he was told that his behavior was "totally out of control and unacceptable." In response he screamed, "I'll kill you!" as he threw a plastic pitcher of water at a staff member.

Changes in Mr. Callahan's Care

When most staff members working with Mr. Callahan followed Don's approach, there were fewer troubling incidences of Mr. Callahan's difficult behaviors. However, changes in work assignments and replacements due to staff turnover led to new staff replacing those who had developed good working relationships with Mr. Callahan. At this point, there was again an increase in the frequency and intensity of Mr. Callahan's challenging behavior.

Still, whenever Don served as Mr. Callahan's nursing assistant, there were no extreme episodes of his difficult behavior. Although Mr. Callahan tended to behave in a grumpy, insistent manner, the intensity of this behavior was generally mild and occasionally moderate. This was the case even when Don's work schedule changed to various times of the day or night.

When Don was not there, periodic, severe episodes of Mr. Callahan screaming insults and threats continued. Staff members working with Mr. Callahan at those times described him as behaving in ways that should not be tolerated, such as constantly insulting, demanding, and threatening them. They said that he was randomly and unpredictably violent. The staff's approach in these cases was to tell Mr. Callahan that he could not speak to them with disrespect, and that his behavior would not be tolerated. Although it had not yet been made a formal treatment plan, Mr. Callahan was told by some of the staff that he could earn the privilege of attending recreation activities by cooperating during care and not threatening staff members. He was also told that if his behavior did not improve, he would be transferred to a locked psychiatric unit because he was a danger to others.

Some Staff Members' Reactions to Don's Approach

Don explained his approach to Mr. Callahan's difficult behavior to the other staff members. Unfortunately, a number of them said that he was simply being manipulated by Mr. Callahan and that treating him nicely was only rewarding his difficult behavior.

These staff members explained that they thought Mr. Callahan was causing a split in the staff, manipulating some staff members, such as Don, to "enable" his bad behavior while others were trying to properly address it. In their view, Mr. Callahan was trying to undermine the staff's efforts to address his difficult behavior effectively. They insisted that his episodes of difficult behavior could only be improved by clearly telling Mr. Callahan that his behavior was wrong and would not be tolerated, and by setting strong limits on his behavior by enforcing the limits with consequences. Some of these staff members expressed anger at Don for supporting Mr. Callahan and making excuses for his detestable behavior. They were dismayed that Don could not see that Mr. Callahan needed to be stopped.

The staff members who opposed Don most strongly also spoke of feeling burned out because of the abuse they encountered from residents such as Mr. Callahan, someone who really did not deserve the amount of care and attention Don was advocating. This level of stress made them dread coming to work, affecting both the care they provided at the long-term care residence and in their personal lives.

The Treatment Plan for Mr. Callahan

In Mr. Callahan's case, the approach of Don's fellow staff members was formalized into a behavior contract. Don was counseled not to allow Mr. Callahan to split the staff. He was instructed to follow the plan and help the other staff present a united front to Mr. Callahan.

As all staff, including Don, followed the new formal treatment plan, Mr. Callahan's behavior became increasingly aggressive, even with Don. He started throwing objects at staff members and frequently screamed obscenities. Shortly after his new care plan was put in place, Mr. Callahan was transferred to a locked psychiatric unit in response to his escalating difficult behavior.

As part of his treatment plan, Mr. Callahan was then informed that he could earn the privilege of being in an unlocked setting by complying with recommended treatment and eliminating his difficult behaviors. To comply with recommended treatment, Mr. Callahan agreed to begin taking antipsychotic medications aimed at reducing aggressiveness, something he had refused earlier.

Effects of Staff Grievances in the Case of Mr. Callahan

The staff were correct that there was a split among the staff about what should be done in regard to Mr. Callahan's behavior. However, this split was not created by Mr. Callahan. The disagreement about Mr. Callahan's case only brought to light the staff's fundamentally different beliefs about what causes difficult behavior and how best to respond to it.

There was a variety of beliefs about the causes of Mr. Callahan's difficult behavior and about what were the most appropriate responses to it. Some staff believed Mr. Callahan had a mental illness, while others believed this was just an excuse to explain the bad behavior of a mean man. Some said it did not matter whether he had a mental illness or not; his troubling behavior needed to stop. These individuals believed he had a choice in how he behaved and that he should be held accountable for his choices. Others believed that there are right and wrong behaviors and that the only correct response to wrong behavior is punishment. If the behavior continues, the punishment should be increased until the problematic behavior stops, even if this requires administering medication (typically sedating medication), to which the individual objects. All of these various beliefs about the causes of and appropriate responses to Mr. Callahan's behavior were held by staff members who opposed Don's approach.

Don's strategy focused on addressing Mr. Callahan's behavior in a way that reduced his emotional distress and any associated negative health consequences. Staff who supported Don's approach understood the principles of behavior change described in this book:

- Positive reinforcement of behaviors is typically more effective than negative or aversive consequences.

- Adequate assessment of what triggers and reinforces an individual's behaviors includes using approaches such as the ABCs of Behavior (particularly in the interpersonal context) in combination with active listening.

- Lasting behavior change in various situations and relationships is often gradual (especially in long-established behaviors). However, when the correct triggers and reinforcers of a behavior are adjusted, there is usually a notable change in the behavior in a relatively short period.

- Successful goals for behavior change are realistic (that is, the immediate and complete elimination of a challenging behavior that occurs frequently and with significant intensity is unlikely).

- Recognizing, acknowledging, or praising positive behaviors, improvements, and efforts is positive reinforcement of desired behaviors and improvement (providing these is *not* the same as being manipulated).

- Maintaining a genuine, positive relationship with those dependent on care is a central aspect of adequate healthcare, including mental healthcare, and is the responsibility of those providing treatment and care, such as supervisors and the administrators of healthcare, in long-term care settings and programs. Attuned, empathic interpersonal experiences are central to adequate health-care, mental healthcare, long-term care.

The principles and techniques described in this book can be quite effective in reducing or eliminating challenging behaviors and the emotional distress or broader health problems related to them. This is so whether those behaviors are viewed as resulting from mental illness or not. However, as in Mr. Callahan's case, grievances can lead to a focus on the idea that fairness requires that the person with challenging behaviors be held "accountable," rather than working toward realistic goals of simply reducing or eliminating the behaviors by addressing the mental health/behavioral health/stress management needs underlying the behaviors.

Staff who opposed Don's approach felt a particularly strong grievance over how Mr. Callahan treated them. The staff members behind the treatment plan that ultimately led to Mr. Callahan's transfer to a locked unit felt it was only fair that he experience negative consequences for his bad behaviors.

In these situations, accountability often translates into making the offender experience certain negative consequences or punishments. When staff see such accountability as a goal of treatment planning, they may not be as likely to see the principles and techniques presented in this book as being effective. Even when treatment teams and staff describe a treatment plan in terms of withholding "rewards" and consider accountability as treatment rather than punishment, it is important to keep in mind the care recipient's experience of such treatment.

Unfortunately, failure of grievance-influenced treatment plans can often lead a grievance-focused team to insist that more controlling, coercive, and negative consequences are necessary. In such instances, the resident's escalating difficult behavior is seen as justification of the very approaches that are triggering and reinforcing the behavior. At the same time, staff grievances only intensify, creating more stress for everyone involved.

Additionally, staff grievances can lead to an overreliance on a medication-centric approach to addressing challenging behaviors, an approach emphasized in widely disseminated versions of the medical model of care. This approach places medications in the central position of treating challenging behaviors, promoting the view that they are *the* best, or only, real treatment, despite evidence to the contrary. This view remains in the field even in the face of national laws aimed at reducing the overreliance on certain medications (for example, the Omnibus Budget Reconciliation Act of 1987 [OBRA 1987], also known as the Federal Nursing Home Reform Act). This medication-centric view was strongly supported by a number of the staff members who were opposed to Don's approach to addressing Mr. Callahan's difficult behavior.

The formal treatment plan for Mr. Callahan's case became quite different from the one Don would have designed. It was also very different from one that might have been followed had mental health advance directives been put in place for Mr. Callahan.

Don's care of Mr. Callahan showed the positive impact of using the types of strategies outlined in the Essentials of Care section of the Advance Directives: MH/BH/SM Form. In cases where staff are at least somewhat influenced by their grievances, the Essentials of Care section of the form (Handout 5.3) may be useful as part of ongoing education. Once completed by a resident, a resident's next of kin, or a designated healthcare proxy, the Essentials of Care section can be copied and posted in the resident's room, perhaps near his or her bed or in some other easily visible location.

Handout 5.5 shows what Mr. Callahan's Essentials of Care list might have looked like.

We have just looked at how grievances can negatively impact how we provide care and make treatment decisions. Now we will consider a method for coping with the grievances we can experience when we encounter difficult situations in our work.

Forgiveness and Coping with Grievance-Related Stress

Forgiveness can be an effective way to cope with and relieve grievance-related stress. Forgiving someone means that we are choosing to no longer hold that person responsible for the emotional distress we feel. Instead, the process of forgiveness focuses our attention back on ourselves and allows us to recognize our unacknowledged emotional or behavioral reactions to wrongful treatment. It helps us regain, or realize for the first time, our own ability to influence how we feel, which can give us a sense of peace and a greater freedom in how we evaluate and respond to problematic situations. When we use forgiveness to recognize our power over our own emotional distress, we avoid the role of victim and instead become an individual who can overcome challenges and succeed. Practicing forgiveness expands our peaceful moments, an effective way of coping with stress.

Practicing forgiveness does not mean ignoring bad or upsetting events or condoning the hurtful behavior of others. However, it can help us reduce the stress of our reactions to these difficult situations.

Techniques for Practicing Forgiveness

Dr. Fred Luskin is a psychologist whose research has looked at how people can forgive those who wrong them, including people who have been physically or mentally abused and people who lost loved ones to murder or armed conflict. He has written about how those who forgive can benefit from forgiving. The discussion in the sections that follow of techniques for practicing forgiveness are described in his book, *Forgive for Good: A Proven Prescription for Health and Happiness*. Based in his research on forgiveness, Dr. Luskin's book outlines how to put forgiveness into practice. If you have practiced the stress management techniques described in previous chapters of this book, you may find that these forgiveness techniques fit very easily into your continued practice.

Widening the View

When we are significantly stressed, we tend to focus on negatives. Our view narrows, leaving out the positive aspects of situations, events, places, tasks, the past, the future, people. This negative perspective can deepen and perpetuate our stress. It is very difficult to feel happy and healthy when everything seems hopeless, scary, or bad. It is very hard to have positive feelings about others when they seem essentially inconsiderate, rude, insulting, mean, hurtful, or cruel.

However, simple "positive thinking" is not optimally effective because it denies problems or negatives. It is important not to ignore upsetting events or to condone the hurtful behaviors of others. It is also important to spend time reflecting on the positive aspects of your life. Widen your view of your life. When we broaden our perspective in this way, we choose to acknowledge the negatives, but also to see and feel the positives.

When you are preoccupied with a grievance, take time to think about something you enjoy, that brings you comfort and a sense of peace. Refocusing on the positive can be hard when you are immersed in a grievance. However, with practice it gets easier. Recall the simplest pleasures, such as seeing sunlight on the leaves of trees, feeling comfortably snug on a cold day or pleasantly cool on a hot day, smelling a pleasant fragrance, feeling the embrace of someone you love, or seeing others experience joy. When dealing with a grievance, thinking about the good in your life is one way of widening your view and expanding your peaceful moments.

See Handout 5.6 for a review of how to widen your view and realistically see and experience the positives in your life.

The Breath of Thanks

As mentioned earlier, forgiveness is a process that helps us regain or recognize our ability to consciously influence our emotions as a way of reducing the power our grievances have over us. The Breath of Thanks exercise can help expand your moments of peace by empowering you to positively influence your emotions. This is a breathing-focused exercise that takes just a few minutes. Practicing it twice a day may help reduce stress and expand your peaceful moments.

First, allow your breathing to gently push your belly out. Then, feel your belly relax and soften as you exhale. Take three to five breaths in this way.

Continue to breathe naturally and easily, and think of your breath as a gift that you simply receive. As you exhale, silently say "thank you." Notice how good it feels just to breathe. Again, silently say "thank you" as you breathe out. Allow yourself to feel fortunate for the goodness in your life. Think of how you feel when you experience the gift of a gentle breeze, the wonder of a clear night sky, the gentle sounds of a content baby, or the smile of someone you love. You may choose to imagine your feelings of gratitude contained in your heart. This may strengthen the feeling. For a total of five to eight exhalations, silently say "thank you."

Expanding your peaceful moments uses your own influence over your emotions to enhance your ability to prevent the stress of your grievances from controlling your emotions. To review the steps for practicing the Breath of Thanks, see Handout 5.7.

Heart Focus

Another exercise for increasing your power over how you feel is called the Heart Focus. This exercise combines elements of breathing-focused relaxation and mental imagery.

To begin, sit or lie down comfortably and close your eyes. Focus your breathing on your belly, letting your belly effortlessly rise as you inhale. Let your belly relax and soften as you breathe out. Focus on your breathing in this way for about 5 minutes.

At this point, think of a moment when you felt a powerful sense of love for someone. This person should *not* be someone with whom you have a significant grievance. Alternatively, you can focus on a memory of nature's tranquil beauty. If you focus on a moment of love for someone, vividly bring the moment to mind. See your loved one in that moment. Hear that person. Notice any pleasant fragrance. Feel the touch of that person. Re-experience that moment. Remember the aspects of your loved one that filled you with positive emotions, contentment, and peace. These feelings may intensify if you imagine them centered in your heart.

If you choose to think of a scene of natural, tranquil beauty, recall it in detail. Think of the sights, the sounds, the fragrances. Allow yourself to experience the renewal of your sense of comfort, stillness, and inner quiet as you bring the details of the scene to mind. Your sense of peace may grow if you imagine it centered in your heart.

During your practice of this Heart Focus exercise your mind may wander. Other thoughts may distract you. If you notice this is happening, refocus on your breathing. Gently inhale. Gently exhale. Return to your peaceful memory.

After 10–15 minutes of practicing this exercise, open your eyes and continue with your day. Doing this exercise for 10 to 15 minute sessions at least three times a week may expand your moments of peace. Work toward a goal of three 20-minute sessions, for a total of 60 minutes a week. See Handout 5.8 for a list of steps for practicing the Heart Focus exercise.

The Heart Focus and Breath of Thanks exercises work best when you set aside time to practice them. After practicing them as described for a period of 2 to 3 weeks, you may notice an improvement in how you feel throughout your day, not just during your practice sessions. You may find yourself using elements of these exercises as you go through your day, accepting the gift of a breath and recalling a sense of love and peace as you exhale.

Even as you integrate aspects of these exercises into your day, there may still be times when you feel stressed in the heat of a moment. At such times, try using the technique of positive emotion refocusing, which is discussed in the section that follows.

Positive Emotion Refocusing Technique

Dr. Luskin refers to positive emotion refocusing technique as "PERT." A brief exercise that combines breathing-focused relaxation and mental imagery to refocus your emotions during a stressful or challenging situation, PERT can be used at any time and in any place to help you remain calm and cope with stressful grievance emotions.

To utilize PERT, begin by focusing on your breathing when you feel stressed by a grievance or a continuing relationship problem. Consciously let your breath push your belly out. Then, let your belly soften as you exhale. Take two of these belly breaths.

On your third belly breath, mentally visualize a person you love. It should not be someone with whom you have a strong grievance. Alternatively, visualize a place of natural beauty that brings you feelings of awe and wonder. Continue the soft belly breathing.

Perhaps you can imagine that your positive feelings toward the person you love, or the awe and wonder you feel about nature's beauty, are centered in your heart.

Continue your soft belly breathing.

If you feel this sense of relaxation and peace focus in your heart, ask your heart what you can do to resolve the immediate difficulty you are experiencing. If you feel your positive feelings collect in another place or part of yourself, ask that peaceful part of yourself what you can do to resolve the difficulty.

For a quick summary of these steps for using PERT, see Handout 5.9.

Using PERT, the Heart Focus exercise, and the Breath of Thanks can be very helpful in claiming positive power over how you feel. In addition to practicing these exercises, consider the principle behind them—that what we choose to focus on or think about in our day-to-day interactions can have a significant impact on our emotions. If we focus on our experiences of love and beauty instead of stressful events that have hurt us, we will feel more positive, peaceful, and empowered.

The techniques for practicing forgiveness can be very effective. However, finding forgiveness calls on us to further examine how our thinking and feeling are linked to the grievances we feel. The section that follows demonstrates how to adapt the ABCs of Thinking and Feeling into the ABCs of Forgiveness by showing how freeing your emotions and beliefs from grievances can lead to forgiveness.

Thinking, Feeling, and Forgiving Grievances

As discussed in earlier chapters, our feelings and thoughts affect each other. To a significant extent, we are able to change what we feel by altering self-defeating patterns of thinking. How and what we think affects the level of stress we feel.

In Chapter 4, we looked at the ABCs of Thinking and Feeling and how what we think about an event can affect how we feel about that event. In *Forgive for Good*, Dr. Luskin describes a link between our grievances and unenforceable rules, which are examples of "shoulding" (described in Chapter 4). As we discussed in that chapter, shoulding is a common unhelpful pattern of thinking that involves believing that something should or must be a certain way. Like Dr. Luskin's unenforceable rules, shoulding involves rule making: "Mr. Callahan has to (or should) respect me. He must at least behave politely." This is an unenforceable rule. Mr. Callahan could choose to treat me disrespectfully and he might never feel respect for me, no matter what I do to enforce these rules.

To resolve the pitfalls of our unenforceable rules, we can use the ABCs of Thinking and Feeling to exert conscious influence over our feelings. When we do this, we avoid leaving our emotional well-being in the hands of the person who has wronged us and reduce our grievance-related stress.

When our rule, our "should," is violated, we typically take it very personally and feel hurt, or anxious, or angry. We generally respond in extremes, as though we need this person to follow our rule at all costs. When we insist on a rule, such as how Mr. Callahan should, must, or has to treat us with respect, we are likely to feel even more personally attacked and distressed when this rule is continually violated.

Unenforceable rules, or "shoulds," are often associated with a cycle of increasingly stressful reactions and insistence on our shoulds. We may shift our focus from the initial rule to another rule: If the first rule is not followed and cannot be enforced, then the offender must experience a negative consequence for the violation. This rule is based on a particular view of fairness, as we saw in the case of Mr. Callahan: If I have been wronged, hurt, or put out, it is only fair that someone be held responsible and that the responsible person be made to feel similarly. When this rule is broken and we are prevented from providing a negative consequence to the offender, we may shift our focus to another rule: Someone else (often an authority figure) must ensure that the offender feels a negative consequence. An unfortunate aspect of these cascading rules is that the more we try to enforce them, the more likely it is that the offender will see him- or herself under attack and fight back.

However, at times the offender may instead comply, but only temporarily to avoid punishment. In these cases, there is a risk that the previous offenses will be compounded when the offender decides to stop complying and returns to violating our rules. We can become enmeshed in an escalating power struggle as we persist in insisting that our rules must be followed. Such a struggle can be expected to inflict increasing stress on all involved. Frequently, the power struggle continues until the side with the most power uses overwhelming force to restrain, restrict, control, or be rid of the offender. None of these outcomes is desirable in a long-term care residence.

In long-term care, treatment planning to address challenging behaviors can become guided or significantly influenced by shoulding. Unfortunately, the more prevalent this kind of problematic pattern of thinking is in a care setting, the more likely it is that the setting will be a stressful environment. A stress-filled organizational culture is highly unlikely to effectively meet the needs of care recipients or staff.

The more each person working in long-term care recognizes when he or she is engaging in shoulding, the easier it will be to reconsider and re-evaluate the impact of unenforceable rules, or shoulds, on the culture of care.

Recognizing Shoulding Using the ABCs of Thinking and Feeling

One of the first steps to dealing with our grievance-related stress and enabling ourselves to practice forgiveness is to recognize and use our own influence on our thoughts and feelings. The ABCs of Thinking and Feeling is a tool for helping us to recognize when we are using problematic patterns of thinking, such as shoulding.

In order to consciously influence how we feel and how we think, we need to recognize clues that we are stressed. These clues can be intense unpleasant emotions, distressing physical symptoms, loud or curt speech, or unawareness of our emotions. Another clue might be behavior toward another person that is co-ercive, controlling, or punitive. Recognizing these clues is part of the process of identifying the emotional **C**onsequence in the ABCs of Thinking and Feeling.

It is also critical to perceive what event or events appear to trigger our stress, our emotional consequence. Knowing which events trigger or strengthen our distress is identifying the **A**ntecedent in the ABCs of Thinking and Feeling. After recognizing the emotional **C**onsequence that we are under stress (the C) and what events triggered the stress (the A), we can clarify our **B**eliefs (the B) about the event. If we were treated poorly by Mr. Callahan, we might have a number of beliefs about the incident and about Mr. Callahan. Pay close attention to how these beliefs build on each other, and escalate our distress:

- "Mr. Callahan has to treat me with respect."

- "He must not insult or shout at me."

- "If he disrespects me, insults me, or shouts at me, I will feel wronged, hurt, and angry, so he should be made to feel the same way and he should be made to stop. That is only fair."

- "If I can't stop his behavior by showing him that it is unacceptable and won't be tolerated, someone else has to make him stop."

This type of thinking is clearly an example of shoulding and a likely contributor to our emotional consequence of stress. However, just as problematic thinking patterns such as shoulding can compound our stress and interfere with our ability to provide care, our thoughts also have the power to help us decrease our stress. They can help us reduce our grievances, practice forgiveness, and expand our moments of peace.

The ABCs of Forgiveness

Rethinking what we believe about an event can change how we feel. Considering other valid perspectives and interpretations of what happened can help us regain control over our own emotions and contain our grievances. This does not mean that we should strive to completely eliminate any emotional influence that others have on us. Being deeply and meaningfully emotionally connected to others is a vital part of mental and physical health. Conscious awareness of that emotional connection allows us to make choices in our interactions with others that increase the depth and meaning of those enriching connections. Being aware of our emotional connections to others and how they relate to our thinking allows us to consider alternative ways of interpreting negative, emotional events.

This process of considering valid alternative interpretations of interpersonal interactions was discussed in Chapter 4, with the case of Belinda, a nursing assistant. The discussion that follows provides a closer look at Belinda's experience.

We saw how Belinda used the ABCs of Thinking and Feeling in her work with Mr. Putin, a long-term care resident. Mr. Putin yelled insults at Belinda, triggering a strong emotional reaction in her. At first, she did not think she needed to examine her beliefs about what Mr. Putin did. Belinda thought it was obvious that he had no right to treat her that way. She thought to herself, "He should not talk to me like that. He always treats me like filth. He never acts like a human being. No matter what I do for him, he is never satisfied. I get so furious just thinking about it." Then Belinda noticed that the more she concentrated on these thoughts about Mr. Putin and his difficult behavior, the more anger she felt.

Belinda discovered she had an unenforceable rule that no one should speak to her the way Mr. Putin had. She also noted that the more she insisted on this unenforceable rule, the more she engaged in other patterns of thinking that also increased her stressful, angry reaction to Mr. Putin's treatment of her. For example, she labeled Mr. Putin as a nonhuman and overgeneralized her view of him until she interpreted everything Mr. Putin did as an example of his disrespect toward her. She took Mr. Putin's behavior very personally.

However, Belinda noticed that she felt less angry when she focused on other thoughts about Mr. Putin and how he behaved, such as, "Someone who acts this way has learned to expect that he must be abusive to get what he wants or needs. His doing that is more likely to push people he needs away . . . or get them to retaliate. He must expect that I will only pay attention if he is abusive. He doesn't really know me. I make mistakes sometimes, but that doesn't make me a G—d— b—— as he called me. He only acts this way sometimes. Yesterday we joked together while I helped him to bed. Maybe we will tomorrow, too."

Belinda reconsidered her initial beliefs about Mr. Putin and his behavior. As she revised her thoughts, which were based in either-or, all-or-nothing thinking, she felt less bound to her unenforceable rule that no one could speak to her as Mr. Putin had. As she reconsidered her beliefs about Mr. Putin and his behavior, Belinda felt more at peace. She no longer believed that her feelings were completely in the hands of Mr. Putin. She no longer held him responsible for how she felt. That is, Belinda forgave Mr. Putin.

For a quick review of the ABCs of Forgiveness, see Handout 5.10.

Adding a "D" to the ABCs of Forgiveness

As we saw previously, we can expand the ABCs method to include "D," which refers to the step of "Disputing," or questioning, our interpretation of an upsetting event. Following Belinda's example, you can dispute or re-examine your own patterns of thinking that contribute to grievance-related stress.

The following three-step process can be particularly helpful in disputing our shoulds or unenforceable rules. First, look for any of the previously described clues that you are stressed (see Handout 5.4). Second, ask yourself, "Am I insisting or demanding that something be different than it is?" An example response to this question might be, "I am demanding that Mr. Callahan never express himself in rude or insulting ways." Third, rephrase this demand as a wish or hope, such as, "I hope that my interaction with Mr. Callahan will not include his calling me names or criticizing me."

As you convert your demand into a statement about what you hope or wish will happen, another strategy you can use is what Dr. Luskin calls "reconnecting to your positive intentions." This strategy involves refocusing on the positive goals and intentions you had before the hurtful event. After experiencing an emotionally harmful event, ask yourself what you had hoped would happen in the situation. State what your hope was in one or two sentences. State what you wanted the specific positive outcome to be. For example, you might answer, "I hoped to effectively help Mr. Callahan and to have him appreciate me and the help I was giving him." This is the type of positive hope that we might constructively restate as a rule when we are stressed: "Callahan's bad behavior is not to be tolerated. He has to treat people with respect."

When our hoped-for goal is blocked, we typically feel hurt and perhaps nervous and unhappy. We then may respond to those emotions with anger, masking our initial feelings of distress or anxiety. In these cases, when we are only aware of our anger toward the situation, it can be helpful to think back to what our initial positive intention was and remember that with every hope comes the possibility of failure. We cannot make what does not happen, happen. Insisting that one should have such control is another unenforceable rule.

Handout 5.11 includes a summary of steps for re-evaluating shoulds and unenforceable rules. Use Exercise 5.2 to practice these steps.

When you have truly learned to replace insisting and demanding with hoping and wishing, you will feel more of a sense of peace and forgiveness. If you have followed the approach for addressing your unenforceable rules described in this chapter and you do not experience an increase in your positive feelings, it may help you to review Chapter 4 and practice the exercises included there. In addition, it could be helpful for you to review and practice the stress-management techniques in each of the previous chapters. Afterward, return to this chapter's sections on practicing forgiveness as a stress management technique.

Social Support and Coping with Grievance-Related Stress

Talking with one or two trusted people about a grievance you have can help reduce stress by allowing you the chance to articulate what happened and how you feel about it. It allows others to provide you with the kind of social support and guidance that may decrease any sense of isolation or loneliness you might feel.

Such sharing of experiences typically increases a person's general sense of happiness and ability to cope with stress. Regularly having such discussions is also associated with good overall health.

The best social support we receive includes a mix of active listening, honest feedback, and, perhaps, assistance to change. The worst social support remains focused on complaining and wrongly encourages us to resist helpful advice. Unfortunately, when our self-esteem is most fragile, we are most attracted to the less-helpful type of social support. When seeking social support, ask yourself, "Does the support I'm receiving have the characteristics of the most beneficial support? Does it have the characteristics of the least helpful?"

Summary

In Chapter 5, we examined how documented advance directives may provide a better alternative to the common type of behavior contract when addressing the challenging behaviors of care recipients. We considered how documented advance directives might be used to proactively address the mental health, behavioral health, or stress management needs that underlie difficult behaviors.

Finally, we discussed how practicing forgiveness can reduce the grievance-related stress we experience when we are wrongly treated by a care recipient. Here we examined ways to identify that we are reacting to specific grievances and engaging in negative patterns of thinking, such as shoulding. We considered how to empower ourselves to reduce our grievance-related stress by recognizing and claiming influence over our own emotions. When we no longer hold others completely responsible for the hurt we feel, we forgive them—expanding our moments of peace and reducing our stress.

Advance Directives: MH/BH/SM

Part 1A. Statement of my intentions

I _____, being of sound mind, voluntarily provide the following healthcare instructions. I provide these instructions now in case, at some time in the future, I am unable to clearly express my wishes or am unable to make informed decisions due to illness or due to my experience of circumstances that led to a level of stress that interferes with my thinking clearly enough to make informed decisions about my care.

In any stress management or mental health situation that is not covered by this document, I designate _____ as my proxy to make decisions regarding my care if I am unable to think clearly enough to make informed decisions about my care or if I am unable to express my decisions.

Advance Directives: MH/BH/SM

Part 1B. Statement of my intentions

(To be completed by the designated healthcare proxy, or other appropriately designed person, if a mental health, behavioral health, or stress management advance directive has not been documented for _____ _____ prior to the time he/she was unable to think clearly enough to make informed decisions or was unable to express them.)

As the healthcare proxy (or other appropriately designated person) for_____,
I _____ being of sound mind, voluntarily provide the following healthcare instructions. I provide these instructions now in case, at some time in the future, I am unable to express them or am unable to make informed decisions due to illness or due to my experience of circumstances which led to a level of stress that interferes with my thinking clearly.

Statements or requests made in the remainder of this document are often made in the first person (for example, "Please recognize that I am experiencing stress"). Although I am completing this form, these statements or requests are intended to be understood as those of _____
(name of care recipient).

Essentials of Care

Check all that apply.

1___	Listening
2___	Allowing choices
3___	Letting me know that you notice improvements in what I do, even small ones
4___	Letting me know you see my positive efforts
5___	Finding what triggers my stressed behavior, including when interacting with others
6___	Finding what reinforces my stressed behavior, including when interacting with others
7___	Supporting my positive efforts at coping with stress Learning about how I effectively coped in the past
8___	Helping by changing the factors external to me that trigger or reinforce my stressed behavior
9___	Recognizing and responding to my need for attention
10___	Avoiding arguing, making repeated demands, or scolding
11___	Avoiding labeling my stressed or challenging behavior as "unpredictable" or "unprovoked" (see items 7 and 8)
12___	Giving me space and time to calm down
13___	Recognizing signs of your own stress when dealing with mine Taking care of yourself is important
14___	If my behavior remains very stressed or challenging, or becomes more so, consulting with others who have found effective ways of dealing with similar situations

Signs of Grievance-Related Stress

To respond most effectively to grievance-related stress, it is important first to recognize that we are under such stress.

Clear Signs: Clear signs involve our strong and/or persistent troubling emotions of which we are aware. We are aware that they are triggered and/or reinforced by our having been poorly, wrongly, or cruelly treated by someone. These emotions can include irritation, frustration, anger, rage, anxiety, fear, terror, unhappiness, sadness, depression, and despair. A mix of such feelings in response to being mistreated is typical.

Apparent Signs: With apparent signs, we do not (but could, if we thought about it) recognize the link between our distress and the way we were treated. Here we can have a vague sense of stress; physical problems, such as headaches or upset stomach; general worsening of physical conditions (seek appropriate healthcare for these); and feeling emotions such as those listed above.

Unacknowledged signs: When we are unaware of having particular emotions or stress related to how we are treated, we can have unacknowledged signs of stress. Some common unacknowledged signs include staying overly busy with tasks or activities; withdrawing from others; being generally inclined to insist, demand, or argue; feeling a sense of indifference, a sense of "objective" detachment when poorly treated; or feeling emotionally numb.

Essentials of Care

Check all that apply.

1 X	Listening
2 X	Allowing choices
3 X	Letting me know that you notice improvements in what I do, even small ones
4 X	Letting me know you see my positive efforts
5 X	Finding what triggers my stressed behavior, including when interacting with others
6 X	Finding what reinforces my stressed behavior, including when interacting with others
7 X	Supporting my positive efforts at coping with stress Learning about how I effectively coped in the past
8 X	Helping by changing the factors external to me that trigger or reinforce my stressed behavior
9 X	Recognizing and responding to my need for attention
10 X	Avoiding arguing, making repeated demands, or scolding
11 X	Avoiding labeling my stressed or challenging behavior as "unpredictable" or "unprovoked" (see items 7 and 8)
12 X	Giving me space and time to calm down
13 X	Recognizing signs of your own stress when dealing with mine Taking care of yourself is important
14 X	If my behavior remains very stressed or challenging, or becomes more so, consulting with others who have found effective ways of dealing with similar situations

Widening the View

A grievance reaction to being wronged is stressful. Typically, such a reaction leads us to focus on negatives. We can come to think that negatives are more real than positives. Hurt or angry feelings can seem more true, more to be trusted than good, warm, or peaceful feelings.

However, to reduce your stress it is important to allow positive, peaceful experiences into each day. They are no less real or true than painful experiences of hurt and anger.

Each day allow yourself to take a broad view. See not only the bad things in your life, in others, and in the world, but also see or experience such things as:

- A breeze brushing across a field of tall grass

- The sound of waves on the shore

- A sunrise

- A sunset

- A cool drink when you are thirsty

- The fragrance of trees and flowers

- A hug

- A smile

- A laugh

- A friend

Source: Luskin (2003)

The Breath of Thanks

This breathing-focused exercise can help you to deepen your experience of the good in your everyday life. After you practice it twice a day for at least two weeks you may find that it assists in expanding your moments of peace.

First, notice your breathing. Feel your belly as it gently, effortlessly pushes out when you inhale. Feel your belly relax and soften as you exhale.

Second, notice how good it is just to breathe. Think of your breath as a gift that you simply receive. Silently say "thank you" as you exhale.

Third, allow yourself to feel fortunate for the goodness in your life, in your day. The goodness may be in the gift of such things as a gentle breeze, the wonder of a clear night sky, the gentle sounds of a contented baby, or the smile of someone you love.

Fourth, imagine that holding in your heart the feeling that you are fortunate may strengthen the feeling.

Say "thank you" this way for 5 to 8 exhalations.

Source: Luskin (2003)

Heart Focus

Using this exercise may help you strengthen your ability to skillfully influence how you feel, reduce your stress, and increase your moments of peace.

First, sit or lie comfortably. Close your eyes. For about 5 minutes, each time you inhale, allow your belly to gently and effortlessly rise. Each time you exhale, let your belly relax and soften. As you continue breathing this way, go to the second step.

Second, bring to mind one of the following:

- A moment in which you felt a powerful sense of love for someone. This should not be someone with whom you currently have a grievance.

- A memory of nature's tranquil beauty.

Vividly bring to mind the sights, sounds, feel, and fragrances of the experience with your loved one or with nature. When your mind wanders, refocus on your breathing and return to your memory of love or beauty.

Third, imagine that centering the feelings of love, contentment, tranquility, or peace within your heart may increase and strengthen the feelings.

You may notice that your general stress level has decreased after about 2 weeks of practicing this exercise, if you:

- Practice 3 days a week

- Practice at least 10–15 minutes on days you practice

- Practice for a total of 60 minutes each week

Source: Luskin (2003)

Positive Emotion Refocusing Technique (PERT)

This exercise may be most helpful after you have practiced other stress management exercises, such as those based in breathing-focused relaxation and mental imagery, for at least 2 weeks.

During, or just after, a situation in which you were treated wrongly:

1. Breathe by letting your breath gently push out your belly. Let your belly relax and soften as you gently exhale.

2. On your third exhalation, do one of the following:

   • Visualize someone you love. This should not be someone with whom you currently have a grievance.

   • Visualize a scene of awe-inspiring natural beauty.

Continue belly breathing.

3. Imagine that the positive feelings of love or awe are centered within and around your heart, to strengthen the feelings.

4. Wherever your positive feelings are centered in your body (perhaps your heart), ask that part of yourself, "What can I do to resolve this difficult experience?"

Source: Luskin (2003)

The ABCs of Forgiveness

Our grievance reactions to being wronged are stressful. Signs that we are having a grievance reaction to being treated poorly, rudely, or meanly may include unpleasant emotions such as anger, anxiety, or feeling down; physical symptoms such as a racing or pounding heart, muscle tension, fatigue, or headaches; feeling detached, indifferent, or numb; tending to insist, demand, or argue; avoiding or withdrawing from others; and withholding things others may feel a need for and may be entitled to.

A. Our grievance-related stress reactions are caused by an **A**ctivating event in which we experience being hurt or wronged by someone.

Belinda, a nursing assistant, was helping Mr. Putin into bed when he said, "You're a G__ d___ b____!"

B. **B**eliefs are our thoughts about the event and why it happened.

First, Belinda thought, "He can't talk to me that way. He always treats me like filth. He never acts like a human being. No matter what I do for him, he is never satisfied."

Later, Belinda thought, "Someone who acts this way has learned to expect that he must be abusive to get what he wants or needs. He must expect that I will only pay attention if he is abusive. He doesn't really know me. I make mistakes sometimes, but that doesn't make me a G__ d___ b___ like he called me. He only acts like this sometimes."

C. We experience emotional **C**onsequences to what we think or believe about how we were treated.

Belinda realized that the more she thought about Mr. Putin in a negative way, the more intensely angry and stressed she felt.

Later Belinda noticed that she felt better, less stressed, when she did not overly personalize Mr. Putin's behavior. She saw that the behavior was caused by other factors than just her interaction with Mr. Putin. She acknowledged that Mr. Putin acted in difficult ways sometimes, rather than holding on to the belief that he always treated her like filth and never acted like a human being.

Re-evaluating Shoulds and Unenforceable Rules

When we think that something should or should not be a certain way, we are likely insisting on an unenforceable rule. Insisting that something should or should not happen when it does happen typically leads us to have stress reactions.

To reconsider "shoulds" or unenforceable rules:

1. Notice signs that you may be experiencing stress: strong unpleasant emotions; physical problems, such as headaches, muscle tension, worsening medical conditions (consult a healthcare professional as necessary); feeling detached, indifferent, or numb; or behaving toward others in negative ways, such as arguing, demanding, withdrawing, withholding, avoiding.

2. Ask yourself, "What am I demanding be different than it is?" Clearly state the answer to this question. For example, you might respond, "No one can talk to me like that!

3. Convert your statement of your demand into a statement of hope. What were you hoping for? What were you wishing would happen? For example, you might say, "I was hoping to do my job well and have it be appreciated."

Recognizing when we have turned our hope or wish for a situation into an unenforceable rule generally helps us to reduce our stress. It allows us to avoid power struggles and helps us to address problems flexibly and creatively.

Source: Luskin (2003)

EXERCISE 5.1

Note: This exercise may be best done individually rather than as a group. However, when done as part of a class or workshop, it may be helpful to have a discussion of participants' experiences of, or reactions to, doing the exercise.

Think of an incident in which someone in your care treated you rudely, poorly, wrongly, hurtfully, or cruelly. If you cannot think of an incident involving a person in your care, think of one involving someone else. Briefly describe what that person did that was rude, mean, hurtful, or cruel. Be specific about what he or she said and did in treating you poorly.

During and/or after the incident:

What emotion did you have that you recognized as being clearly related to the way you were treated? (check all that apply): __none; __irritation; __frustration; __anger; __rage; __anxiety; __fear; __terror; __sadness; __ depression; __despair; __other
(specify _____

_____

_____

_____

_____)

During and/or after the incident:

Which of the following did you experience, *although you did not see the emotion(s) as being linked to how you were treated wrongly?* (check all that apply): __a vague sense of stress; __physical problems, such headaches or upset stomach; __general worsening of physical condition(s); __ emotions such as those listed above; __nothing; __other
(specify _____

_____

_____

_____

_____)

(continued)

During and/or after the incident:

Which of the following did you experience while not having, or being unaware of having, any emotional reactions to the incident? (check all that apply): __feeling indifferent; __a sense of "objective" detachment; __emotional numbness; __increased involvement with tasks or activities; __withdrawal from others; __increased inclination to insist, demand, argue, or fight; __over-eating; __drinking alcohol/using drugs; __other (specify _____

_____

_____

_____

_____)

If you checked any of the above items, you may have experienced stress related to being treated rudely, poorly, wrongly, hurtfully, or cruelly. These items are frequent indicators of the need for managing the stress we experience. Recognizing them as possible indicators of stress can be a first step in doing something about the stress.

EXERCISE 5.2

Think about an incident in which you were rudely, poorly, wrongly, or meanly treated by a care recipient. Think of an incident involving someone else if you cannot think of one involving a care recipient.

Briefly describe the incident.

What signs were there that you were stressed at the time of the incident or shortly after it? These signs might include strong unpleasant emotions; physical problems, such as headaches, muscle tension, or worsening medical conditions; feeling a sense of indifference, numbness, or "objective" detachment; or behaving toward others in ways such as arguing, demanding, withdrawing, withholding, or avoiding.

What do you think the other person did that should not happen or must not happen or that is unacceptable, not to be tolerated, or not allowable? Clearly state the answer to this question. For example, you might say, "No one can talk to me like that," "No one should be allowed to treat another person that way."

Convert your insistence about what "should" be into a statement of hope. What were you hoping for? What were you wishing would happen? For example, you might answer, "I was hoping to do my job well and have it appreciated."

CHAPTER 6

Obstacles to Using Effective Techniques

This chapter looks further at the obstacles we encounter when trying to address challenging behaviors in the most effective ways. Obstacles to using the principles and techniques described in this book can take at least three forms: personal, institutional, and societal. Personally, we may not know about or be familiar enough with them. Institutionally, the policies or usual practices of a long-term care setting or program may interfere with providing attention to the needs underlying the difficult behavior. Finally, a society that tends to undervalue people who are older or ill will not devote the necessary time, money, or other resources to meet their needs.

Although much of this chapter addresses obstacles confronted by staff and administrators in institutional settings or programs, those who provide care outside of these formal settings will still likely find the basic material in this chapter useful and relevant.

Chapter 6 ends by further describing how good relationships with others can help us cope with stress and presents ways to improve our interactions and relationships with others to help us manage stress.

Personal Obstacles

By this point, we know some of the key strategies and techniques for reducing or eliminating challenging behaviors. However, we may still need to practice and apply the skills that are most likely to reduce or eliminate challenging behaviors. We may also have set ideas about ourselves and others that prevent us from using the best approaches to address difficult situations with those in our care. The following beliefs can be personal obstacles to providing the best care:

- A person's behavior should change if you tell him or her that the behavior is unacceptable.

- Using only negative consequences will teach someone to stop a difficult behavior.

- Some behaviors are just plain bad, and anyone who engages in them does not deserve respect.

- Trying to understand a challenging behavior is just making excuses for the behavior and blaming others.

- Nothing that one person does affects the way another person thinks, feels, or behaves, especially if that person has a mental illness, dementia, or a difficult personality.

- Some people do things for no reason.

- Someone who does bad things is just a bad person.

- People do not change.

Another group of beliefs that are likely to impede our developing skills is related to responsibility, authority, and power. Some of these beliefs include:

- It is not my job or responsibility to deal with difficult behavior.

- A care recipient should be made to stop behaving in insulting, verbally abusive, or threatening ways.

- It is the responsibility of those in authority to make people stop engaging in challenging behaviors.

Coping with Our Personal Obstacles

A first step toward dealing with personal obstacles is recognizing them. If the difficult behavior of the person we are caring for does not improve or gets worse, this can be a strong clue that personal obstacles are present. While it is important to address any medical conditions contributing to the difficult behavior, lack of improvement in behavior can be a sign that we need more training or supervision in the techniques described in this book. Consulting with a qualified mental health professional, taking classes, studying, and getting supervision can all help us to improve. Generations of mental health professionals have found that their own participation in personal psychotherapy greatly enhances the effectiveness of their work. Participating in therapy may be beneficial to anyone who works in long-term care, too. In addition, nonprofessional caregivers are also likely to benefit from therapy. It can be helpful in dealing with stress and in making significant improvements in one's ability to effectively deal with challenging behaviors.

Psychotherapy typically entails meeting with a psychotherapist on at least a weekly basis. In addition to being effective treatment for depression and anxiety, therapy can help with substance abuse, family and relationship problems, and with specific work-related difficulties. Psychotherapy can also be a useful tool in helping us better recognize and respond to our own needs and those of others.

Some people have health insurance policies that cover much of the cost of psychotherapy. Universities sometimes have psychological services offered to the community at low or no cost. State or county psychological associations typically are able to make referrals to therapists, including those whose fees are adjusted according to an individual's ability to pay.

Consultation with a mental health professional about a particular person's behavior will probably result in the recommendation to use methods similar to those presented in this book. The mental health professional may also give some suggestions about how to use the techniques more effectively. It is not likely that the mental health professional will take responsibility for addressing the care recipient's challenging behavior. Successfully addressing the challenging behavior of someone who is dependant on others for care requires the efforts of each person involved in that care or contributing to that care environment.

It is usually not helpful to insist that a person in authority be the one to stop a care recipient's challenging behavior. Relying on force, intimidation, threats, restraints, or negative consequences does not promote emotional or physical health or improved behavior.

Primarily authoritarian approaches to difficult behaviors do not encourage exercising, maintaining, or developing a care recipient's sense of competence, self-control, or self-worth. Such approaches are more likely to encourage or intensify the individual's experience of frustration, resentment, anger, and depression, all of which can motivate additional challenging behaviors.

Challenging behaviors are signs of psychological distress. Consultants, supervisors, and administrators in long-term care settings or programs have important roles in creating an environment that promotes care recipients' general well-being, including their psychological well-being. However, providing care for the individuals' psychological well-being is a central part of *everyone's* job in long-term care settings, not just those in authority. See Handout 6.1 for a summary of potential personal obstacles to addressing challenging behaviors.

Institutional Obstacles

Supervisors and administrators can significantly influence how a long-term care setting operates. The policies and procedures that they support affect a facility's or program's values and goals. Their style of leadership also has a major impact on what others in the long-term care setting do.

Long-term care communities, in particular, commonly emphasize certain tasks and policies that make it difficult for staff to use the most effective techniques for dealing with residents' challenging behaviors. An overemphasis on the physical and medical tasks and interventions performed by staff can overshadow the psychological tasks and interventions needed to promote residents' well-being. Clearly, it is very important to ensure that residents get needed medications, are clean, have clean bedding and clothing, and are fed. However, exclusively or persistently prioritizing completion of these tasks, over the social interactions with residents during and after such tasks, can lead to significant behavior and overall health problems, even if physical and medical needs are met. Problems arise when factors that make interactions positive are considered unnecessary or beyond what's expected of staff members, especially if attending to these factors requires more time and effort than staff, managers, or administrators think they should expend.

Another institutional emphasis that can cause problems is using the minimal amount of resources needed to provide care—that is, the minimal numbers of qualified staff to accomplish the "real" physical tasks. Not having a workable approach to retaining staff is also a frequent problem. Working in a long-term care setting involves complex interpersonal, organizational, and task skills, many of which develop through experience and training. High staff turnover prevents the cultivation of skilled staff members.

Leadership style in long-term care communities and programs can also affect how well difficult behaviors are addressed. A primarily "top-down" approach relies on telling staff what to do rather than helping them develop skills they can use responsibly and creatively. This approach stresses giving orders and emphasizes doing tasks to avoid negative consequences from authority figures. It focuses staff attention on the power of supervisors rather than on flexible and creative ways to address the challenges of their work.

Addressing Institutional Obstacles

Job descriptions for all the personnel of long-term care facilities and programs must clearly state that addressing the mental health, behavioral, or psychological needs of care recipients is a central part of each job position. New employee orientation can underscore this crucial aspect of long-term care work. Appropriate job descriptions would also outline staff members' responsibilities for participating in ongoing training and supervision aimed at reducing difficult behaviors or satisfying psychological needs. Supervisors and administrators can support staff members' learning by modeling effective approaches with care recipients. Because the techniques described in this book apply to many situations and relationships beyond those involving care recipients, supervisors and administrators can also model these approaches with other staff members.

Continuing education and supervision, including peer supervision, in the use of the techniques and principles described in this book are essential for supervisors and administrators. Peer supervision might take the form of groups of supervisors or administrators meeting to discuss issues related to addressing challenging behaviors.

Those who facilitate the development of a long-term care setting's policies and practices also have the responsibility to ensure that ongoing training and supervision are available for all staff. It is important to recognize that training and supervision sessions are not helpful when staff members do not have time away from direct resident care. Scheduling policies can give staff time to attend training sessions, to focus during supervision sessions, and to use the techniques described in this book.

It also is not helpful to train staff in techniques that are difficult or impossible to practice because of workload demands. In some instances, it may be necessary to reassess standards used to determine adequate numbers of staff. For example, it may not be realistic to expect a nursing assistant who helps 13 or more residents with most activities of daily living to be readily available for training and supervision or to be able to carry out the best practices for addressing residents' psychological, behavioral, or mental health needs.

Guidelines for staffing or consultation by other disciplines and occupations are also critical. For example, recreation therapists, psychologists, psychiatrists and other medical staff, social workers, rehabilitation staff, housekeepers, clerical staff, dietary personnel, and clergy all contribute to the optimal functioning of a long-term care community. Each of these disciplines and occupations focuses on critical aspects of the overall well-being of residents, and no one discipline (for example, nursing) can reasonably assume full responsibility for these aspects.

Attending to adequate staffing and consultation can enhance job satisfaction among staff and help reduce staff turnover. Another strategy for retaining staff is to adopt a democratic style of leadership. This approach encourages staff to develop their abilities to work both creatively and cooperatively, generating solutions to challenges and working together toward a shared mission. With this type of leadership, the mission of the long-term care setting emphasizes creating an environment—through relationships with those in need of care—that is sensitive and responsive to residents' physical, psychological, and other needs. Enhancing staff members' roles requires supervisors and administrators to be open to insights and feedback from all staff, and also calls for leadership in facilitating the process of shared decision making and implementing resulting decisions that are consistent with the facility or program's mission.

The democratic style of leadership values each person, as well as his or her capacities and contributions. This style of leadership is very different from the authoritarian style described previously. The authoritarian style may have short-term benefits: staff may do what they are told, when they are told to do it, and how they are told to do it. Typically, though, staff under this type of leadership will do little else. They tend to be less creative in solving the many challenges that confront them when the leader is not present or for which the leader has not left specific orders. In addition, groups with authoritarian leaders are prone to unconstructive conflict, arguing, and fighting.

A third type of leadership is the laissez-faire approach. Supervisors and administrators who use this hands-off style avoid providing guidance and facilitating processes aimed at addressing challenges or accomplishing goals. Instead, they leave staff members on their own. Unfortunately, this style usually leads to very little being accomplished. It is not likely to address care recipients' difficult behavior or psychological needs.

To address the institutional obstacles that come from authoritarian or laissez-faire leadership styles, supervisors and administrators can work on developing more democratic leadership skills with ongoing team-building processes and programs. Team building requires open communication (promoted by active listening skills); acknowledgment of the important roles and contributions of team members (promoted by praise and compliments); respect for each person's independent work (promoted by allowing choices); cooperative problem solving (based on understanding that problems have triggers and, if they continue, have reinforcers); and a sense of a shared mission (meeting the needs of those receiving long-term care). As these points illustrate, integrating this book's basic techniques and principles into a long-term care staff's daily interactions with care recipients and other staff members constitutes a significant step in the process of team building.

One final issue regarding institutional obstacles is selecting people for leadership and staff positions in long-term care facilities. Selecting people for positions for which they are not well suited can be a significant obstacle to the practice of the skills and principles described in this book. Not everyone is prepared to practice the necessary basic skills required in long-term care settings. How people are selected would most appropriately rely on knowledge of what is needed to do the work well, as well as what characteristics of a job applicant best predict that the person would be successful in the position. The selection process would be aimed at finding a good fit between the person hired and the job for which he or she is hired to perform. There are human resource firms that have expertise in designing such selection processes. There are also universities that have programs that train industrial/organizational psychologists who have expertise in creating these selection processes. Such university programs can be good resources for long-term care organizations that have an interest in ensuring the best possible care for those they serve.

See Handout 6.2 for a review of ways to address institutional obstacles.

Societal Obstacles

The functioning of a long-term care facility or program is also affected by the wider society. Society's general attitudes about long-term care communities, for example, influence whether a long-term care community's services are valued. Widely held opinions, beliefs, and feelings about aging, elderly people, disabilities, disease, and death influence the amount of attention and resources society devotes to long-term care communities.

Our society tends to value youth over age. There are widespread negative beliefs about aging. Examples include the belief that people's personalities change in negative ways as they age and that all older people are depressed. In fact, negative changes in personality and major depression are the exception among older people. Although depression is more common among long-term care community residents than among older people in the wider community, depression can generally be treated successfully in long-term care settings with adequate resources.

Responding to Societal Obstacles

Familiar people, places, and situations are often less likely to frighten us. Learning more about unfamiliar people, places, or events can help us confront and work through our negative perceptions and fears. Long-term care communities and programs can help the broader society to confront its negative perceptions and fears of aging, elderly people, disabilities, disease, and death by strengthening ties with the community in order to promote familiarity with their facilities and programs. They can develop and deepen relationships with religious and volunteer or service organizations as well as educational institutions—from child care centers to graduate and professional schools. The aim is to deepen and broaden connections between the people of the long-term care world and those of other organizations.

Long-term care facilities and programs can sponsor cultural, educational, and entertainment events for those they serve as well as for staff, members of other organizations or institutions, and the general community. Interaction and dialogue among people from these different groups can provide the long-term care facility or program with valuable feedback about how the facility and its residents are perceived, as well as ways to improve those perceptions. See Handout 6.3 for a summary of how to overcome societal obstacles.

A System View

We as individuals, long-term care institutions and programs, and the wider society together form a system. As parts of the system, the individual, the institutions and programs, and the society interact with and influence each other.

It may seem impossible to change institutional, social, or even individual attitudes or policies that have a negative impact on how we provide care. However, the acts of individuals do affect the acts of others. The more positive our influence as individuals is, the better the odds are that improvements will happen within our care settings and beyond. To some degree, the techniques described in this book for addressing difficult behaviors can be used in our individual interactions with everyone in the long-term care world. We do not have to wait for institutional or social change to use these approaches: listening, allowing choices, praising and acknowledging, cooperative problem solving, the ABCs of Behavior, the ABCs of Thinking and Feeling, the ABCs of Forgiveness, engaging in positive relationships with others, and more generally taking good care of ourselves by managing our stress. The more we use these techniques and basic principles, the more we will contribute to improvements in the care environment.

Improving Relationships as a Stress Management Technique

Stress is part of life. We are challenged to meet everyday demands. Our personal obstacles to coping with stress may mesh with obstacles put in place by our institutions and society. It can take practice to change our less-constructive responses to stress. In addition to engaging in regular exercise and using the stress management techniques previously described, we can focus on building positive relationships. Our relationships play an important role in helping us manage stress.

We have examined ways of striking a better balance between the stress of everyday life and the relief of pleasant activities and relaxation. Recall the list of pleasant events featured in Handout 1.2 of Chapter 1. You may have noticed that many of these activities involve other people. That is because positive interactions and positive relationships with others play an important role in helping us reduce stress, cope with unavoidable stress, and maintain or improve physical and mental health. In addition to engaging in other types of pleasant activities and relaxation practice, effectively coping with stress typically requires regularly spending time and communicating with at least one other person. This person should be someone you can talk to about yourself, about your life, and about what you think and feel. With this person, you can talk about both good and troubling things. When you talk with this person, you feel accepted, respected, and liked (or loved). This is not the kind of relationship that you have with everyone. It is a special, close relationship.

Typically, a balance between being open to others expressing themselves and expressing ourselves deepens relationships and helps us cope with stress better. Mutual give-and-take relationships are the most beneficial. These are relationships in which each person generally feels listened to, heard, and accepted. They are also relationships in which each person feels a good deal of freedom to express thoughts and feelings. Some people are better at establishing and maintaining this type of relationship than others. It may not be possible to surround yourself with only people who are good at forming give-and-take relationships, but it is best to put limits on the number of relationships in which you give more than you get.

Relationship Skills

Much of this book deals with interactions between people—that is, interactions that form the basis of relationships. The heart of the book is about how relationships play a fundamental role in determining how those we provide care to behave, think, and feel. Many of this book's techniques can be used in your relationships with people other than those in need of long-term care. For example, others will generally be more open to hearing what you think and feel if you regularly use active listening with them.

Another way to foster rewarding relationships is to let people know what you like about what they do. Be descriptive in praising or complimenting them. A good general rule: For every negative comment or criticism that you give someone, give the person at least four genuine compliments. It is good to express your appreciation for little qualities or actions, not just the big ones. Examples include "I notice that you carry your neighbor's recyclables out to the curb for him. That's a very caring thing to do," or "Thanks for listening to me talk about how tough things have been at work lately. Talking it out with you helped me get some relief," or "I'm glad that you can talk to me about what's going on in your life." Notice effort, too, not just the final product. For example, you could say, "It was very good of you to try to straighten up the house before I got home."

Expressing Yourself

Each of us is likely to express some feelings and thoughts well and others not well at all. We are also probably more skilled at expressing ourselves with some people than with others. However, developing our ability to express ourselves well can help deepen and strengthen our relationships and general social skills. See Handout 6.4 for examples of common situations in which people have difficulty expressing themselves.

Passive, Aggressive, and Assertive Communication

There are three general styles of expression: passive, aggressive, and assertive. If your usual style is passive, you typically do not say what you feel or think about what others do, or you tend to be indirect and apologetic when you do express your feelings and thoughts. An unfortunate result is that others are likely to treat you as though what you think and feel does not matter. An example of passive communication involves Jack letting his daughter Melanie borrow his car. Melanie returned the car after the time Jack needed it to get to work. When Jack got into the car, he found that the gas gauge was on empty. He did not tell Melanie that these inconveniences bothered him. In fact, when Melanie asked to borrow the car again the next day, Jack said, "Sure, it's just sitting in the driveway."

If your style is usually aggressive, you are most likely to express yourself in ways that force others into paying attention to you and what you think or feel. What you say often tells people that they are stupid or worthless for not seeing matters the way you do, not treating you the way you want to be treated, or not doing the tasks you think they should. It tells others that what you want, feel, and think is more important than their own desires, feelings, and thoughts. For you, it is important to come out on top in your dealings with others. Here is an example of aggressive communication using the previously presented situation: Melanie returned the car late and with nearly no gas. Jack said, "I can't believe you! You are so self-centered! Everything is about you, isn't it?! What you want. 'Gimme, gimme.' 'I want this. I want that.' You're selfish. You disgust me!"

When your style is assertive rather than aggressive or passive, you are generally able to say what you think and feel without disregarding or disrespecting yourself or others. You do not usually communicate in ways that are hurtful or humiliating. Assertiveness is most likely to build strong, beneficial relationships. Building on the same case, here is an example of assertive communication: When Melanie returned the car late with the gas gauge on empty, Jack said, "When I lent you my car, I got it back late and there was almost no gas in it. I felt angry because I had to get to work and I was going to be late."

Assertive communication uses "I-messages," which tell what happened as you see it, how you feel about what happened, and why you feel that way. They often begin with the phrases, "What I think is . . . ," "What I feel is . . . ," "The way I see the situation is . . ." I-messages do not focus on blaming, labeling, attacking, counterattacking, threatening, telling people "You can't get away with that," humiliating people to put them in their place, or showing others who is boss.

Most people respond well to assertive communication. However, some will not. They will retreat as though attacked, perhaps acting hurt and withdrawn. Others might react with hostility to counter what seems to them to be an attack. When others have such negative reactions, use active listening and other ways of encouraging their positive behavior toward you. If such negative reactions are usual for someone you are obligated to live, work, or deal with, it can be good to regularly use active listening skills and other ways of supportively encouraging positive behavior.

Do not let relationships with those who frequently have strong negative reactions to your needs dominate your life. Set limits to the amount of time, energy, and effort you spend in such relationships. Setting limits can help you avoid getting overly stressed or burned out. Balance the stressful effects of these relationships by spending time with others who are better able to see, hear, and accept you. Spend some time at least once per week with someone who is able to accept you in this way. To review guidelines for assertive communication, see Handout 6.5. Practice applying assertive communication in your own life with Exercise 6.1.

Setting Limits

Setting limits in a relationship means putting limits on what you are going to do for, tolerate from, invest in, or give to the other person. We set limits on what we will or will not do in response to the other person's behavior. We avoid trying to set limits on what the other person does because trying to control others does not usually lead to the best outcomes. It is generally better to encourage the person's cooperation and self-control by using the techniques described in this book.

If limit setting becomes your primary way of interacting, it is not likely to be very effective. In addition, if the other person routinely responds to limit setting with rage or withdrawal and helplessness, continuing to emphasize limit setting may not be the best approach. When you are persistently setting limits or are avoiding setting any limits, you are probably in an ongoing power struggle or are feeling hopeless. In either case, you and the other person are not having your basic needs met for attention, acceptance, positive regard, and control. If these needs are not fulfilled in the relationship, it is best to have other relationships in which they are. If these needs are not met for someone who depends on your care, it is important to have that person's care provided by someone else until you are less stressed and are able to accept that responsibility.

Limit setting can be illustrated by recasting the story of Jack and Melanie. In this scenario, Jack stated the limit by clearly telling Melanie that she could use the car as long as she returned it on time and with a full tank of gas. Jack told his daughter that if she brought the car back late or without a full tank of gas, he would know that Melanie chose not to be allowed to borrow his car for a week. Jack put a limit on what he would do (lend his car) and what he would tolerate (having his feelings and needs disregarded or abused). He also pointed out that Melanie had the choice of whether she would be able to borrow the car in the future.

Melanie returned the car late but with a full tank of gas. Jack acknowledged the positive by saying it was good of her to have filled the tank. However, he followed through with the limit of not lending his car to Melanie for a week because the car was returned late. He said, "It was good of you to fill the tank, but I see that you have chosen—by returning the car late—not to borrow the car for the next week." Melanie was angry, replying that he was unfair and ruining her plans. Jack said, "You're disappointed and angry because you can't borrow the car for a week," and left it at that. The next time Jack lent Melanie the car, she brought it home on time and with a full tank of gas. In the future, Jack planned to continue following through with the limits he set on lending his car.

For guidelines and practice on setting limits in your own life, see Handout 6.6 and Exercise 6.2.

Summary

Chapter 6 examined personal, institutional, and societal obstacles to using the most effective ways for addressing care recipients' difficult behaviors. Various suggestions were given for coping with these obstacles. We can practice recognizing the obstacles that we as individuals put in our own way. Such obstacles can be overcome through education, training, and supervision and perhaps psychotherapy. We also need to keep in mind that challenging behaviors are signs of psychological distress and that providing care for the psychological needs of care recipients is part of the job for everyone working in a long-term care setting, as well as for everyone accepting the role of caregiver for those dependent on care. Yet, we can recognize that certain policies and practices of a long-term care setting or program may impede the psychological tasks and interventions that are necessary for a healthy, safe environment. A democratic style of leadership as well as developing and deepening relationships with organizations and institutions outside of long-term care settings can help address both institutional and societal obstacles. Even if institutional or societal change has not occurred, it is important to use the techniques described in this book. Despite institutional or societal obstacles, our individual actions can lead to needed improvements in long-term care.

Chapter 6 ended by discussing the importance of good relationships in managing stress. It explained how expressing ourselves well can deepen and improve relationships. In addition, the chapter described ways of limiting exposure to stress in difficult situations and relationships.

Working on Personal Obstacles to Using Effective Approaches to Residents' Difficult Behaviors

Personal obstacles can impede using the best techniques for dealing with care recipients' challenging behaviors. We can take the following steps to address these obstacles:

Recognize that if medical conditions have been addressed and the behavior persists or worsens, a significant part of the problem could be that you may need to know more about, or increase your skill in using, effective principles and techniques for addressing the behavior.

Consult with a qualified mental health professional, attend classes on dealing with the psychological needs and difficult behaviors of those in your care, and/or get supervision on these topics. Generations of mental health professionals have found that their own participation in personal psychotherapy greatly assists the effectiveness of their work. Therapy would likely be helpful for those working in long-term care as well. It can help address difficulties we have in our work and our relationships. Psychotherapy is generally effective treatment for problems such as depression, anxiety, and substance abuse. It can help us better recognize our own and others' needs and how best to respond to them.

Understand that difficult behaviors are signs of psychological distress. Each person working in long-term care shares responsibility for meeting care recipients' needs, including the psychological needs that can motivate difficult behaviors. These needs can be met by practicing the basic techniques of addressing challenging behaviors.

Reducing Institutional Obstacles to Using Effective Approaches to Difficult Behaviors

Institutional obstacles are the policies or practices in long-term care that limit use of the basic principles and techniques for addressing difficult behaviors. Long-term care supervisors and administrators can work on such obstacles by applying these guidelines:

Helpful job descriptions for all personnel in long-term care settings clearly state that providing care for the mental health and behavioral or psychological needs of care recipients is a central part of every position. They state the expectation that all staff members will develop proficiency in the basic techniques for addressing residents' psychological needs and dealing with difficult behaviors.

Selection for leadership and staff positions should be done by identifying the best fit between applicants and positions. Not everyone is well suited for every job. Human resources firms and university Industrial/ Organizational Psychology programs can be resources in designing selection processes.

New employee orientation can provide an overview of recognizing signs of psychological distress, such as difficult behaviors, and the basic principles and techniques for dealing with them.

Because the basic techniques are interpersonal skills, they are helpful in any relationship. **Supervisors and administrators can model the use of these skills** in dealings with others, including staff and residents.

Ongoing training and supervision in the use of basic principles and techniques is important for all staff, supervisors, and administrators.

Staff members need enough time away from direct patient care to regularly attend training and supervision sessions; therefore, appropriate scheduling and staffing policies are necessary. Having adequate numbers of staff also ensures that one's workload does not make using the basic principles and techniques too difficult.

(continued)

Reducing Institutional Obstacles to Using Effective Approaches to Difficult Behaviors

Cultivate a leadership style that values each person's contributions— a style that helps others develop skills and encourages the creative and cooperative use of those skills. This democratic leadership style promotes open communication and responds to feedback and suggestions that will help the long-term care setting fulfill its mission. This style facilitates a team approach to accomplishing the goals of an organization or program.

Keep the primary mission of long-term care in mind: to provide an environment, through relationships with those in need of close attention and care, that is sensitive and responsive to care recipients' physical, psychological, and other needs.

Working on Societal Obstacles to Using Effective Approaches to Residents' Difficult Behaviors

Negative views of long-term care facilities and unpleasant preconceptions of elderly people—related to fears of illness, disability, and death—can undermine the broader society's support for and involvement in long-term care facilities. These fears, along with our society's largely youthful orientation, can prevent the investment of enough time, money, and other resources to enable long-term care facilities to meet the needs of residents. Long-term care facilities can help members of society confront and work through negative perceptions and fears by promoting ways to become more familiar with the world of long-term care. Familiarity can lead people to question their preconceptions. Some ways of encouraging this familiarity are as follow:

Develop and deepen relationships with religious, volunteer, service, and educational organizations (from child care centers to graduate and professional schools).

Sponsor entertainment, cultural, and educational events that are open to and involve long-term care residents and staff, members of other organizations or institutions, and the community.

Look for feedback from members of the different groups that interact with the long-term care facility about their perceptions of the facility and its residents and about ways of improving those perceptions.

Common Situations in Which People Have Difficulty Expressing Themselves

Turning down a person's request to borrow something of yours

Asking for an expected service when it was not offered

Asking a favor of someone

Resisting sales pressure

Expressing a different opinion from the person(s) with whom you are talking

Expressing your love to someone

Asking to borrow something

Telling someone how you feel when he or she has done something unfair to you

Admitting ignorance

Turning down an invitation

Resisting an unfair demand from someone important to you

Asking for constructive criticism

Telling a friend or co-worker that something he or she has said or done bothers you

Asking for clarification when you are confused

Asking a person who you do not know and who is annoying you in public to stop doing something (e.g., playing loud music on a train)

Asking if you offended someone

Telling someone that he or she disappointed you

Telling someone that you like him or her

Criticizing your spouse or partner

Complimenting someone

Source: Lewinsohn, Munoz, Youngren & Zeiss (1986)

Using Assertive Communication in Relationships

Using assertive communication generally helps us effectively express ourselves to others. When we use an assertive communication style, we clearly state what we think and feel. It can often reduce or prevent stressful interactions, may help improve difficult relationships, and may deepen and strengthen positive relationships.

Assertive communication involves using I-messages to say what happened as you see it, how you feel about what happened, and why you feel that way. I-messages are not focused on proving who is right or wrong. When we use I-messages we do not disregard, disrespect, or apologize for our own thoughts or feelings. We simply state them.

Examples of I-messages	Examples of common, usually unhelpful alternatives (either passive or aggressive)
"When you shout at me, I feel frustrated because I want to get along with you."	"I can't stand when you shout. If you shout again, I'll really give you something to shout about."
"You returned my car late. I felt very stressed out. I had to get to work, and I did not want to be late."	"You're such a self-entered jerk."
"I have a lot to do right now. I feel a bit overwhelmed because even though what you're asking me to do is a small thing, I don't feel like I can take on anything else just now."	"I have so much to do that I can't get everything done on time. But I'm sorry. I'll make the photocopies right now that you want for your meeting next week—just as you asked."
"You listened to me talk about what I was going through when I was having a tough time. I'm so grateful. It helped me feel that I was not alone."	Not saying anything.

Most people respond well to assertive communication, but some view it as an attack. They may react by acting hurt and withdrawing or by becoming hostile. When others have negative reactions to your assertive communication, use active listening skills, acknowledge their positive behaviors, and let them make choices in addressing problems. Balance the stressful effects of these relationships by spending time with others who are better able to see, hear, and accept you. Spend some time at least once per week with someone who is able to accept you in this way.

Setting Limits in Relationships

To reduce and prevent some stress, it is important to set limits on the time, energy, and effort we put into difficult interactions and relationships. We set limits by deciding what we will or will not do for, to, or with others—*not* by trying to control their behavior. Although limit setting influences the behavior of others, it is about taking care of ourselves.

Describe the limit calmly. For example, say, "If you scream at me again, I will leave the room. Then I won't talk to you again until dinner."

Act on the limit calmly. For example, say, "You just screamed at me. I see you have chosen for me to leave the room and not talk with you until dinner." Then leave the room. You could also just leave the room without saying anything.

Remember that the most effective limits are mild. They do not deprive or threaten to deprive anyone of safety, basic needs, or fundamental human rights. An example is telling a resident in a long-term care residence that if he or she insults you again, you will leave him or her safely alone for 15 minutes or find a co-worker to provide the care. Never threaten something as severe as leaving the resident confined to bed all day for insulting you.

Remember that limit setting is most effective when it is not the main focus of your dealings with anyone and when it does not result in rage or withdrawn signs of helplessness. If you are either constantly setting limits or not setting any limits, you are likely in an ongoing power struggle or are feeling hopeless. Both you and the other person are not having your basic needs met for attention, acceptance, positive regard, and control. If these needs are not met in this relationship, you need other relationships in which they are. If these needs are not being met for someone who depends on your care, arrange for that person's care to be provided by another person until you are less stressed and are able to accept that responsibility.

EXERCISE 6.1

Think of a time when you were talking with someone at home, work, or elsewhere and had trouble saying what you thought or felt. You may want to refer to Handout 6.4 for examples of common situations in which we have trouble expressing ourselves. Perhaps you had trouble with speaking at all or with speaking without putting the other person down.

Briefly describe the following:

1. What happened

2. How you felt about what happened

3. Why you felt the way you did

Describe "I-messages" that you used, or could have used, to express yourself in this situation.

EXERCISE 6.2

Think of a time when you felt overwhelmed by what someone else wanted from you or when you felt that someone was taking advantage of you, neglecting you, or treating you disrespectfully.

Briefly describe what the person was doing.

Explain how you described, or could have described, the limits you would set if the mistreatment happened again.

Describe how you followed through with, or could have followed through with, the limit you described.

CHAPTER 7

Treatment Planning

Although not used in all long-term care settings, treatment plans are common and can be useful methods for addressing challenging behaviors. This chapter provides guidance in developing successful treatment plans. Readers who are not involved in settings where treatment plans are used may still find aspects of the approaches described here useful.

The basic techniques for addressing difficult behaviors described throughout this book (for example, active listening, allowing choices, using praise) are vital to the first often-overlooked step in the treatment planning process: prevention. The best treatment for difficult behaviors is a preventive approach. If we routinely use these techniques as we interact with care recipients, challenging behaviors are likely to be less frequent and less intense. However, when our attempts at prevention do not work, we need to use more active treatment planning.

This chapter describes two methods of treatment planning: individual and team. In the individual method, the planning process is relatively informal. It occurs when a caregiver uses the approaches described in this book to develop a therapeutic relationship with the care recipient—a relationship that helps to prevent or address difficult behaviors. The team method is required when individual efforts need additional support or guidance. While the team method approach has much in common with the individual method, the planning is formalized and typically occurs during interdisciplinary team meetings.

These methods should be used as flexible guidelines to treatment planning, taking into account the varying needs of different settings and care recipients. However, if you do modify these methods and do not see improved behavior, it may be best to return to following the suggested methods more closely.

The Individual Method

An individual caregiver begins treatment of a care recipient's difficult behavior by deciding how to respond. In some cases, the best treatment is to ignore the behavior. This approach is most effective for infrequent behaviors or actions that are frequent but not harmful (for example, talking to oneself, grumpiness, complaining, infrequent angry outbursts, occasional strong language). Ignoring such behaviors does not mean ignoring the needs that are motivating the behaviors. It means avoiding responding to the behavior by openly showing anger or annoyance, reprimanding the person receiving care, or instructing that person about more appropriate behavior in the heat of the moment. Frequently, such responses reinforce the difficult behavior.

Behaviors that hurt someone emotionally or physically are problematic. They can be harmful to the person engaging in the behavior or to someone else. Examples of such behavior are frequently shouting or screaming, persistently insulting others, making physical or verbal threats, hitting, pinching, biting, kicking, and scratching. These behaviors require caregivers to use an active therapeutic approach. In instances when the behavior poses an immediate risk of significant harm to anyone (including the care recipient), follow your setting's policy for dealing with such situations. This may involve calling a crisis team or even the police.

With the individual approach to treatment planning, a realistic goal is to reduce the frequency or intensity of the challenging behavior, or both. (See Handout 3.4 for a refresher on setting realistic goals.) If you choose to focus on reducing the intensity of a difficult behavior, Handout 7.1 includes a helpful scale to measure the intensity of a difficult behavior. Using this scale, a challenging behavior that is very strong would be scored a 5. In such cases, a realistic goal could be to reduce the intensity to less than 5.

The individual method of treatment planning has five steps, and each takes approximately 2 weeks. At the end of each step, assess the situation. If there is no improvement in the challenging behavior, if it has worsened, or if additional improvement is needed, it is time to move on to the next step.

Each step in this method builds on the previous step. As you move from one step to the next, continue to practice all of the techniques from the previous steps. The steps are outlined in the following sections. For a complete overview of different handouts relevant to each step, see Handout 7.2.

Step 1: Review and Use the Basic Techniques

Review and practice the following basic techniques for the next 2 weeks:

- Keep in mind that the challenging behavior is likely to have both internal and external causes (Handout 1.1).

- Use active listening (Handout 2.1).

- Engage in cooperative problem solving (Handout 3.6).

- Allow the care recipient to make choices (Handout 2.2).

- Use praise and other social reinforcers to encourage positive behavior (Handout 2.3).

- Contain your reactions to the person's behavior (Handouts 2.4 and 3.2).

- Use stretching techniques to address disruptive attention-seeking behavior (Handout 3.5).

Assess the situation after using Step 1 for 2 weeks. If there is no improvement in the behavior, if it has worsened, or if additional improvement is needed, it is time to move on to Step 2.

Step 2: Look for Triggers and Reinforcers of the Behavior

If the basic techniques outlined in Step 1 were not successful, take a closer look at the difficult behavior, observing for potential triggers and reinforcers of the behavior. The goal of Step 2 can still be to reduce the behavior's frequency, intensity, or both or it may be to shorten the duration of episodes of a particular challenging behavior. As you look for triggers and reinforcers to the difficult behavior, continue to use all of the basic techniques from Step 1.

For Step 2, do the following for 2 weeks:

- Use the ABCs of Behaviors to find at least one probable trigger or reinforcer of the behavior (Handouts 3.1 and 3.3).

- Use the ABCs of Behavior Observation Form in the appendix to help you find probable triggers and reinforcers of one or two difficult behaviors. Remember that the triggers and reinforcers frequently lie in how our uses of the techniques in Step 1 are not tailored well enough to fit the needs of the individual.

- Fill in the appropriate section of the form each time you see the behavior happening for up to 2 weeks or until you have an idea of the likely triggers and reinforcers. Infrequent behaviors might require more than 2 weeks.

Step 3: Change the Triggers and Reinforcers of the Behavior

In Step 3, the goal of the treatment plan may still be to decrease the behavior's frequency, intensity, or both or to decrease the duration of episodes. As always, continue using the basic techniques from Step 1 and continue tracking the difficult behavior with the ABCs of Behavior Observation Form as you did in Step 2.

Based on your findings from using the ABCs of Behavior Observation Form in Step 2, your approaches to the problem might include changing the antecedent to the behavior to avoid triggering it, changing the consequence to the behavior to avoid reinforcing it, or changing both. If you have not found any possible triggers or reinforcers, perhaps the behavior happens too infrequently. You may also need to review and practice applying the ABCs of Behavior approach by rereading Chapter 3.

Step 3 also includes using the ABCs of Thinking and Feeling to help you manage the stress of working with the person (Handouts 4.1–4.4). Track these ABCs with the ABCs of Thinking and Feeling form in the appendix. Review the common motivations behind the difficult behavior as you use the ABCs of Thinking and Feeling (Handouts 4.6 and 4.7).

If you see improvement after implementing Step 3, great! Keep up the good work. If there is no positive change, if the problem has gotten worse, or if additional improvement is needed, go on to Step 4 of the treatment planning process. Step 4 concentrates on improving and expanding your use of stress management techniques.

Step 4: Manage Your Stress

Step 4 involves using the stress management techniques outlined in this book to help manage your reactions to difficult behaviors. At the same time, the goal may still be to decrease the behavior's frequency, intensity, or both or to decrease the length of the behavioral episodes.

As always, continue to use and fine-tune the basic techniques listed in Step 1. Also, continue to use the ABCs of Behavior and ABCs of Thinking and Feeling Observation forms from Steps 2 and 3.

In Step 4, do the following for 2 weeks:

- Make at least one more change to the apparent triggers or reinforcers of the difficult behavior. This change would be based on your use of the ABCs of Behavior and active listening.

- Review the handouts on stress management techniques to help you manage the stress of helping the resident with the difficult behavior (Handouts 1.2, 2.5, 3.7, 4.8, 5.5–5.11, 6.4–6.6). Try at least one new technique you have not used before.

If improvement occurs after using Step 4, wonderful! Pay attention to what has been helpful, and give yourself credit for your work. Keep using what you have learned about the resident, about yourself, and about approaches that benefit you and the resident. If there has been no improvement or if the problem has gotten worse, it is time for Step 5.

Step 5: Others as Resources in Assessment

Step 5 involves gathering information from other people. Remember that it is a good idea to talk with your supervisor or a consultant throughout the treatment planning process when you are working with someone with challenging behaviors. It can be very valuable to talk with other caregivers about how they approach the care recipient. It is important to hear from staff members who have not had the same difficult experience of this person. Therefore, as a general rule, in a long-term care setting talk with at least five other staff members to find out about their interactions with the individual and their ways of addressing the person's behavior. When you hear about others' experiences with the person who behaves in a challenging way, pay close attention to how they interact with the person rather than to such things as the staff members' gender, race, or age. Such characteristics are not likely to be the only factors that trigger or reinforce the person's positive or negative behavior.

It might even be helpful to watch staff members interact with the care recipient when that person's behavior is less difficult. Paying attention to what these individuals do can help you learn beneficial and different ways of working with the resident.

For a review of the individual method to treatment planning, see Handout 7.3.

Supervisor's Role in the Individual Method

A supervisor can play an important role in the individual treatment planning process. Actively listening to the staff member is a vital part of this role. Other aspects of the supervisor's role include using praise, compliments, and other social reinforcers to acknowledge and encourage the staff member's efforts and successes, allowing the staff member to make choices, and using cooperative problem solving with the staff member. In addition, the supervisor upholds the mission of long-term care to provide an environment that is sensitive and responsive to the needs of those who require care, including psychological needs, by supporting relationships between staff members and care recipients.

Furthermore, it is important that employee evaluations assess familiarity with the basic skills outlined in this book for addressing challenging behaviors. Supervisors themselves should also be evaluated. The appendix contains a Basic Psychological Skills Evaluation Form, which can be used as part of routine, periodic performance evaluations of personnel.

If there is little success in treating a care recipient's challenging behavior, the supervisor should be mindful that at least one person caring for the individual is probably struggling with using this book's principles and techniques. There are several steps a supervisor can take in such a situation, many of which involve closer supervision of the staff member. One possibility is individual supervision sessions with the staff member, focusing on the use of the techniques. It may be helpful to discuss this book one chapter at a time during supervision sessions. It can be important to let the staff member describe how using the techniques has or has not been effective in different situations with different people. This gives the staff member a chance to consider concrete ways of using the techniques and to think of ways he or she might use the techniques more successfully.

The supervisor can also ensure that scheduling policies allow the staff member to attend training on addressing difficult behaviors. He or she can work on removing institutional obstacles to the staff member's ability to attend such training opportunities.

Another tool a supervisor can use is the buddy system. Using this approach, a supervisor can assign a staff member who is having trouble using the basic techniques to work with another staff member who has been more successful and perhaps has been on the job longer. Allowing staff members to mentor each other in areas in which they have strengths acknowledges and encourages important skills for working effectively in long-term care settings.

If training and supervision do not efficiently help a staff member work well with a particular care recipient, it is best not to schedule him or her to work with that person. With continued supervision, training, and personal growth (perhaps including psychotherapy), the staff member may develop the skills necessary to work with similar care recipients in the future.

In some cases, a staff member's personal obstacles will prevent him or her from effectively using the best approaches in particular situations, despite available training and supervision. For example, a staff member with a history of sexual abuse may not work well with male residents with dementia who expose themselves. Sometimes, a supervisor will be aware of such personal information about a staff member, but often not. This staff member may eventually work through the issues underlying the personal obstacles. However, this process may not happen quickly enough for the staff member to work well with a significant number of residents. When possible, supervisors should assign such staff members to other duties that make better use of their strengths. When reassignment is not possible, the supervisor and staff member might jointly explore the staff member's other employment opportunities and what help he or she may need during the process of seeking new employment.

When a care recipient's challenging behavior is persistent and is a significant difficulty for staff members in general, it is time for the team method of treatment planning.

The Team Method

When a resident's challenging behavior is raised as an issue to be addressed by his or her formal, written treatment plan, the interdisciplinary treatment team serves an important function. This team usually includes members from different areas of expertise, such as physical medicine and rehabilitation, nutrition, chaplain services, internal medicine, social work, psychiatry, dentistry, nursing, and psychology. The team members can discuss their own experiences in working with the resident and can use active listening with each other. In addition, the members can acknowledge, show appreciation for, and offer praise and other social reinforcers for each other's ways of interacting with the resident that are in line with the long-term care facility's mission. They can discuss the basic techniques for addressing difficult behaviors, the best ways to implement them, the potential obstacles to using them, and ideas for overcoming the obstacles. As a general rule, the team can also follow steps similar to those for the individual method to develop and document a treatment plan for challenging behaviors.

Like the individual method of treatment planning, the team method has five steps and each step takes approximately 2 weeks. At the end of each step, reassess the situation. If there is no improvement in the challenging behavior, if it has worsened, or if additional improvement is needed, it is time to move on to the next step.

Each step in this method builds on the previous step. As you and your team move from one step to the next, continue to practice all of the techniques from the previous steps. The following sections outline the steps for this method.

Step 1: Review and Discuss the Basic Techniques as a Team

As with the individual method, the goal of Step 1 is to decrease the behavior's frequency, intensity, or both or to shorten the duration of episodes of a challenging behavior. Team members should review together and use the following basic techniques:

- Keep in mind that the challenging behavior is likely to have both internal and external causes (Handout 1.1).

- Use active listening (Handout 2.1).

- Engage in cooperative problem solving (Handout 3.6).

- Allow the care recipient to make choices (Handout 2.2).

- Use praise and other social reinforcers to encourage positive behavior (Handout 2.3).

- Contain emotional reactions to the person's behavior (Handouts 2.4 and 3.2).

- Use stretching techniques to address disruptive, attention-seeking behavior (Handout 3.5).

- Have realistic goals (Handout 3.4)

In Step 1, treatment planning team members receive the handouts outlining each technique listed above. These are copies of the handouts listed in Step 1 on Handout 7.2. The person who distributes the handouts facilitates a review and brief discussion of their content. The following can be used as discussion questions for the team:

- "How might this handout's suggestions help—or not help—address the resident's challenging behavior?"

- "What are your reactions to this handout's suggestions?"

- "How have these or similar ideas and techniques been helpful to you in other situations with different people?"

- "Why might these techniques be difficult to use, and how can we address these difficulties?"

For more discussion questions, see Handout 7.4.

Encourage team members to discuss their thoughts and reactions to the content of the handouts. Team members might not all agree with everything presented, but discussion can help deepen understanding of the psychological principles and techniques presented in each handout. Team members can also practice their active-listening skills with each other during this discussion.

This process of review and discussion helps treatment team members improve their own as well as other team members' understanding and use of the principles and techniques of addressing difficult behaviors. This team discussion process can also be counted toward the long-term care setting's requirements of ongoing training for staff.

In this step, supervisors or other designated individuals give the handouts describing the Step 1 techniques to staff members who work with, or may work with, the resident but who are not on the treatment planning team. When supervisors or others distribute the handouts, they briefly review them with staff, allowing as much discussion of the material as possible. This is a good time to use active listening, praise, and other social reinforcers with staff members in ways that support the basic mission of the long-term care facility or program. The discussion can include the types of questions previously mentioned for use with the treatment planning team.

Use the techniques of Step 1 for 2 weeks. At the end of the 2 weeks, if there is no improvement, if the behavior has worsened, or if further improvement is needed, move on to Step 2.

Step 2: Identify Triggers and Reinforcers of the Behavior as a Team

Step 2 involves taking a closer look at the difficult behavior by looking for potential triggers and reinforcers of the behavior. The goal of Step 2 can still be to reduce the behavior's frequency, intensity, or both or it may be to shorten the duration of episodes of a particular challenging behavior. As you look for triggers and reinforcers to the difficult behavior, continue to use all of the basic techniques of Step 1.

As a team, discuss the ABCs of Behavior (Handouts 3.1 and 3.3), using the discussion questions in Handout 7.4. Then, use the ABCs of Behavior Observation Form in the appendix for a 2-week period to find possible triggers and reinforcers of the challenging behavior. Each episode of the difficult behavior should be reported to the charge nurse or other designated person who completes the ABCs of Behavior Observation Form, using Handouts 3.1 and 3.3 as guides. It is important for the charge nurse or other designee for completing the form to keep in mind that triggers and reinforcers frequently lie in how our uses of the techniques in Step1 are not tailored well enough to fit the needs of the individual. Clarifying such triggers and reinforcers with staff requires sensitivity to both the needs of the caregiver and the needs of the care recipient, using the same skills that we are encouraging staff to master.

As part of Step 2, supervisors or other designated individuals also discuss the ABCs of Behavior and distribute Handouts 3.1 and 3.3 to staff members who work with or may work with the resident but who did not attend the treatment planning meeting. In this step, the handouts are briefly discussed with staff. This step contributes to ongoing education, training, and supervision. Again, in these discussions make sure to use active listening techniques as well as praise and other social reinforcers with staff members. Encourage staff to make choices in using the techniques that support the basic spirit of the treatment plan.

Step 2 is done for 2 weeks. By the end of this 2-week period, the behavior may improve. If not, or if the behavior has gotten worse or additional improvement is desirable, it is time for Step 3.

Step 3: Change the Triggers and Reinforcers of the Behavior and Manage Your Reactions

Step 3 involves using the information gathered from Step 2 to change apparent triggers and reinforcers of the challenging behavior and manage staff reactions to the behavior. Even if possible triggers or reinforcers have not yet been found, the team should go ahead with the rest of Step 3. Again, the goals continue to be to reduce the behavior's intensity, frequency, or both or to reduce the duration of behavioral episodes. Team members continue to use the basic techniques from Step 1.

Using information from the completed ABCs of Behavior Observation Form, revise some approaches of the treatment plan in order to change triggers, reinforcers, or both. Follow this revised treatment plan for the next 2 weeks. At this point, team members should also pay closer attention to managing their own reactions to the resident and to staff, and consider how to help staff members with recognizing and managing their reactions to the care recipient. During a team meeting, review the ABCs of Thinking and Feeling. As part of this step, each team member receives photocopies of the handouts listed in Step 3 of Handout 7.2. The meeting facilitator or another designated team member leads a review and brief discussion of each handout. See Handout 7.4 for questions that can be used to further the review and discussion.

Part of Step 3 is ensuring that staff members who work with or may work with the care recipient but who are not on the interdisciplinary treatment planning team receive the handouts, too. Immediate supervisors or other designated individuals distribute these, review them with staff, and facilitate brief discussions. Again, see Handout 7.4 for questions to ask that can help in the review and discussion of the handouts. This kind of discussion can be a very important way of providing necessary supervision in addressing difficult behaviors.

If the behavior improves during the 2 weeks of Step 3, wonderful! Congratulations are in order for the direct care staff and the rest of the team. If there has been no positive change, if the problem has gotten worse, or if additional improvement is desired, go on to Step 4 in the team treatment planning process.

Step 4: Manage Stress

Step 4 involves reviewing as a team the stress management techniques outlined in this book. In addition, it invites team members to consider how such techniques may or may not be useful for themselves. This step also calls for the team to facilitate getting stress management information to the staff as part of the treatment planning process. During Step 4, the goal is still to reduce the challenging behavior's frequency, intensity, or both or to shorten episodes of the difficult behavior. The team continues to fine-tune the basic techniques from Step 1 and use information about triggers or reinforcers of the behavior from the observation forms to revise approaches to the problem.

To review and facilitate discussion of the stress management techniques from this book, the meeting facilitator or another designated person distributes photocopies of the handouts listed in Step 4 of Handout 7.2. These handouts focus on a variety of exercises for managing stress and expanding peaceful moments during the workday. Supervisors or other appropriate individuals also provide these handouts to the staff members who work with the care recipient. The person distributing the handouts leads a brief team discussion about the handouts' content and reminds team members to review previously received handouts. The same type of discussion is held with other staff members who work directly with the resident. The questions for reviewing and discussing handouts in Step 1 can be used again here.

If there has been improvement after the 2 weeks that Step 4 is used, great! The efforts of the team and direct care staff have paid off. If further improvement is desirable, the team should use what it has found in the treatment planning process to set new goals and then adjust the approaches as needed. If there still has been no improvement or the behavior has gotten worse, however, the team should go on to Step 5.

Step 5: Identify and Change Root Causes

Step 5 calls for the team to discuss possible root causes of obstacles to effectively addressing the resident's challenging behavior. Root causes are practices or policies that interfere with preventing or implementing solutions to problems. A root cause is any process that prevents what is needed from being obtained. The goal of looking for root causes is not to blame any particular person for problems; rather, it is to identify what organizational, institutional, or societal practices, policies, procedures, or processes contribute to unwanted outcomes or interfere with desired outcomes.

In this discussion, team members focus on what is needed to most effectively provide essential care that addresses the care recipient's difficult behavior. Are there any resources or changes to care that are deemed necessary but that are unavailable in the long-term care setting? Is there any process that prevents what is needed from being obtained?

Sometimes team members may not discern any root causes, but it is helpful for them to at least list what is needed to ensure that the essentials of care are provided in addressing a challenging behavior.

Following the team's discussion of root causes, ideas about what is needed and possible obstacles to obtaining what is necessary can be raised in dialogue with the long-term care setting's administration. In addition, during this dialogue it can be helpful for the team to present ideas about what steps, practices, procedures, or resources are required to begin addressing the obstacles. Such dialogue can lead to an approach to addressing the obstacles, an approach that can be followed in a flexible manner and that is responsive to feedback from staff, care recipients and their families or significant others, and the wider community. To be most effective, this approach would be guided by the mission to provide care that is based in responsive relationships between those in need of care and the people and institutions charged with providing care. See Handout 7.5 for a summary of the team approach to treatment planning.

Summary

This chapter described treatment planning for challenging behaviors. Two methods of treatment planning were discussed: an individual approach that can guide individual staff members in addressing challenging behaviors, and a team approach that can be used when the individual approach does not sufficiently address a care recipient's behavior. Both approaches have five steps, and each step is based on previous chapters of this book.

Finally, this chapter discussed prevention as an approach to the treatment of challenging behaviors. An ongoing process of familiarizing or re-familiarizing yourself with the techniques and principles presented in this book can aid in creating or supporting a long-term care culture that is effective in preventing or limiting the intensity of many difficult behaviors.

Setting Goals for Addressing Challenging Behaviors

It is important to set goals when trying to help a resident reduce or eliminate a challenging behavior. One measurable goal could be to reduce the estimated average number of times the behavior happens during one shift (for frequent behaviors) or during one week (for less frequent behaviors). Another goal could be to shorten episodes of the behavior. For example, if a resident typically yells for 20 minutes at a time, the goal might be that the resident will, on average, yell for less than 20 minutes.

Yet another goal could be to reduce the intensity of the behavior. Using the following scale, the goal could be to reduce the intensity of a behavior scored 5 to a 4 or less. Once a goal has been reached and maintained, set a goal for further improvement, if needed.

Challenging Behavior Intensity Scale

Score and intensity level	Examples
1 Very Mild	A resident tells a caregiver to go away. A resident speaks loudly or sharply but does not shout.
2 Mild	A resident periodically calls for help (without shouting) when there is no significant need for help. A resident sometimes complains using strong language.
3 Moderate	A resident shouts but does not scream. A resident angrily shakes his or her fist at someone. A resident lightly slaps someone's hand.
4 Strong	A resident screams and may also perhaps use ethnic, racist, or gender slurs. A resident vigorously hits someone.
5 Very Strong	A resident scratches someone, breaking that person's skin. A resident hits and bruises someone.

Handouts from *Caring for People with Challenging Behaviors* to Use for Individual and Team Treatment Planning

This list presents the handouts from *Caring for People with Challenging Behaviors* to be used for each treatment planning step.

Step 1

Handout 1.1. Understanding Causes of Challenging Behavior

Handout 2.1. Active Listening

Handout 2.2. Allowing Choices

Handout 2.3. Using Praise, Compliments, and Acknowledgment

Handout 2.4. Things to Avoid When Trying to Encourage Positive Behavior

Handout 3.2. Holding On: Dealing with Reactions to Challenging Behaviors

Handout 3.4. Realistic Goals for Challenging Behaviors

Handout 3.5. Stretching

Handout 3.6. Cooperative Problem Solving

Handout 7.1. Setting Goals for Addressing Challenging Behaviors

Step 2

Handout 3.1. The ABCs of Behavior

Handout 3.3. Determining What Triggers and Reinforces a Challenging Behavior

Review the handouts from Step 1.

Step 3

Handout 4.1. The ABCs of Thinking and Feeling

Handout 4.2. Adding the "D" to the ABCs of Thinking and Feeling

Handout 4.3. Either-Or, All-or-Nothing Thinking

Handout 4.4. Disputing Unhelpful Thoughts or Beliefs

Handout 4.6. Common Motivations for the Difficult Behavior

Handout 4.7. Common Caregiver Reactions to Care Recipients' Difficult Behavior

Review the handouts from Steps 1 and 2.

(continued)

Handouts from *Caring for People with Challenging Behaviors* to Use for Individual and Team Treatment Planning

Step 4

Handout 1.2. Pleasant Events

Handout 2.5. Progressive Muscle Relaxation

Handout 3.7. Mental Imagery

Handout 4.8. Breathing-Focused Relaxation

Handout 6.4. Common Situations in Which People Have Difficulty Expressing Themselves

Handout 6.5. Using Assertive Communication in Relationships

Handout 6.6. Setting Limits in Relationships

Review the handouts from Steps 1, 2, and 3.

Step 5

Handout 5.4. Signs of Grievance-Related Stress

Handout 5.6. Widening the View

Handout 5.7. The Breath of Thanks

Handout 5.8. Heart Focus

Handout 5.9. Positive Emotion Refocusing

Handout 5.10. The ABCs of Forgiveness

Handout 5.11. Re-evaluating Shoulds and Unenforcable Rules.

Review all of the previously listed handouts.

The Individual Method of Treatment Planning for Challenging Behaviors

Step 1: Review and Use the Basic Techniques

Use active listening skills. As much as the resident will tolerate, work with him or her to determine what need motivates the behavior and what can be done about it. Frequently praise any of the resident's positive behaviors and provide the following: smiles, hugs, thumbs-up signs, or pats on the back. Reinforce effort. Remember that behavior change is often gradual. Work toward realistic goals.

Note: If the resident engages in very disruptive attention-seeking behavior, go to him or her often—before the behavior starts. If you cannot reach the resident before the behavior starts, go to him or her before it escalates. Each time you go to the resident, help him or her with the tasks for which assistance is requested, and support the resident's independent efforts, as much as he or she will tolerate. After 1–2 weeks, gradually lengthen the time between your visits—again, as much as the resident will tolerate.

Step 2: Look for Triggers and Reinforcers of the Behavior

After 2 weeks, there may be significant improvement. If the behavior has gotten worse or additional improvement would be helpful, keep using the Step 1 techniques. As you do this over the next 2 weeks, use the ABCs of Behavior to pay careful attention to what happens right before and after the difficult behavior starts so you can uncover triggers and/or reinforcers.

Step 3: Change the Triggers and Reinforcers of the Behavior

Change things that seem to trigger or reinforce the problem behavior. Often, ineffective use of the Step 1 techniques can be a trigger and/or reinforcer. For the next 2 weeks, keep using the Step 1 techniques, but make necessary changes in your use of them to eliminate or reduce triggers or reinforcers. If the behavior happens again, continue to look for triggers and reinforcers.

Note: If you often think that situations and people never change—that they are always bad—you are probably overstressed. Keep in mind that people do not do bad things all of the time, and it is very unlikely that a situation will never change.

(continued)

The Individual Method of Treatment Planning for Challenging Behaviors

Step 4: Manage Your Stress

Adjust one or two possible triggers or reinforcers. Maintain these adjustments over the next 2 weeks. During this time, benefit your work, relationships, and health by taking steps to manage stress. Make sure you take time for yourself every day—time to relax and to do things that you enjoy. Even little things, such as talking with a friend, taking a walk, reading, or sitting quietly, can be important.

Step 5: Involve Others as Resources in Assessment

Talk with your supervisor about your work with the resident's behavior. In addition, talk with co-workers who experience the resident differently than you do. Watch those who have less trouble with the resident for ideas about what you can do.

Note: You can also begin the activities of Step 5 during any of the previous steps.

Discussion Questions

When using handouts as part of the team treatment process or in formal educational settings, it is important to encourage discussion. Use the questions below to promote discussion. Remember to support the use of active listening skills during such sessions; this encourages participants to respond to questions or to raise their own questions regarding the ideas and techniques being considered.

- How might the handout's suggestions help—or not help—address a resident's challenging behavior?

- What are your reactions to the handout's suggestions?

- How have these or similar ideas or techniques helped you in your interactions with residents?

- How have these or similar ideas or techniques helped you in your interactions with other people?

- What made these or similar ideas or techniques effective when you used them with residents or other people?

- What might make it difficult to use these ideas or techniques with residents?

- What can you do to address such factors?

- What else might make it less difficult to use these ideas or techniques?

The Team Method of Treatment Planning for a Challenging Behavior

The treatment planning team reviews and discusses the ideas listed in the following five steps under the direction of the team facilitator or another designated person. The same ideas should also be reviewed and discussed by staff members who work with or may work with the resident and who are not part of the treatment planning meeting. Immediate supervisors or other appropriate people facilitate review and discussion among other staff members.

Step 1: Review and Discuss the Basic Techniques as a Team

Review and discuss listening skills, praise, and other social reinforcers; cooperative problem solving; and—in cases of disruptive attention-seeking behavior—techniques for helping the resident stretch his or her ability to tolerate appropriate intervals without being a focus of attention. In the written treatment plan, note that these approaches will be used to address the resident's difficult behavior. After 2 weeks of following Step 1, move on to Step 2.

Step 2: Identify Triggers and Reinforcers of the Behavior as a Team

Review and discuss how behaviors are triggered and reinforced. Continue to use the techniques from Step 1. Ensure that episodes of the challenging behavior are reported to the charge nurse or other designated person, who notes the behavior as well as what happened just before the behavior occurred, once the behavior started, and just as the behavior ended. After 2 weeks, move on to Step 3.

Step 3: Manage Your Reactions

Review and discuss the importance of managing one's own reactions to the resident. Continue with the techniques from Step 1. Adjust the possible triggers and reinforcers found in Step 2. Update the written care plan to show any adjustments. Continue the search for possible triggers and reinforcers if none have been found yet. Ensure that episodes of the challenging behavior continue to be reported to the charge nurse or other designated person, who records all pertinent details. After 2 weeks, move on to Step 4.

(continued)

The Team Method of Treatment Planning for a Challenging Behavior

Step 4: Manage Stress

Review and discuss additional ways of dealing with one's own reactions to the resident and his or her behavior. As a team, review stress management techniques to help contain emotional reactions to difficult situations. Continue using the techniques from Step 1. Change at least one trigger or reinforcer of the challenging behavior. Note that change on the written care plan. Continue trying to uncover triggers and reinforcers if none have been found yet. Ensure that episodes of the behavior continue to be reported to the charge nurse or other designated person, who records the pertinent details. After 2 weeks, move on to Step 5.

Step 5: Identify and Change Root Causes

If there has been no improvement by this time and the challenging behavior is of strong or very strong intensity (that is, 4 or 5 on the scale presented in Handout 7.1), engage in team discussion of possible root causes (for example, institutional policies or practices encouraged by social standards). Discuss these issues with the administration, and formulate a plan for addressing these obstacles.

Afterword

This afterword is intended for mental health professionals and others who may be interested in further information on the underlying principles upon which the approaches to addressing challenging behaviors described in this book are based.

The basic principles are derived from a tradition of clinical practice grounded in essential elements of the scientific method: observation, documentation, stated hypotheses, tested hypotheses, and replication of results. In fact, *the* fundamental principle upon which the approaches described in this book are based is the clinical application of the scientific method. Here "clinical application" refers to addressing the needs and problems of those we serve in our professional roles. Using the scientific method in this way, as a guide in assessing and addressing the needs of an individual, provides both science-based and person-centered care. This book is the result of various influences from this "real-world" science and from the "laboratory," or academic, approach to science within the discipline of psychology. The discussion that follows describes some of the major influences.

Caring for People with Challenging Behaviors: Essential Skills and Successful Strategies in Long-Term Care largely uses language that is associated with behavioral and cognitive theory and technique (for example, "The ABCs of Behavior" and "The ABCs of Thinking and Feeling"), or the language of cognitive-behavioral therapy (CBT). The language of CBT is clear and direct, well suited to instruction, and a way of directly conveying information in settings such as classrooms, seminars, or workshops or in treatment plans. In further regard to conveying information, the language used in this book is also derived from work in humanistic psychology, which has for decades made significant contributions to providing psychology-informed training materials to various populations. For example, humanistic psychology has promoted awareness of how broadly applicable active listening skills are as tools in helping develop human potential in mental health, parenting, education, and business.

Underlying the use of the language of CBT and humanistic psychology in this book is psychoanalytic theory, research, and practice. Interested readers will find that psychoanalyst Paul Wachtel (1997, 2008) has written exceptionally well about overlap in psychological schools of thought. In particular, he is among those who have demonstrated how aspects of psychoanalysis can be translated into terms that are more closely associated with behavioral and cognitive psychology.

Contemporary psychoanalytic theory, as well as psychoanalytic research and practice, emphasizes the interacting influences of the individual's relational context and the individual's feeling, thinking, behavior, and physiology. The relational world includes the interpersonal and community/societal context as well as the individual's internalized experience of self and others. From a psychoanalytic perspective, whatever diagnosis an individual has, whatever type of personality an individual has, the individual's functioning will be significantly affected by the person's relational context. Most importantly, the individual's experience of interpersonal interactions can trigger and reinforce a range of problematic feelings, thoughts, and behaviors that are often the basis for mental illness diagnoses and that influence and are influenced by other health conditions. Interventions that change the reciprocal influence between the *inter*personal and the *intra*personal can often result in changes in both the relational context and the individual's patterns of feeling, thinking, and behaving. This is the basic psychoanalytic perspective underlying the principles and techniques of *Caring for People with Challenging Behaviors: Essential Skills and Successful Strategies in Long-Term Care*.

Allen-Burge, R., Stevens, A.B., & Burgio, L.D. (1999). Effective behavioral interventions in nursing homes. *International Journal of Geriatric Psychiatry*, 14(3), 213–228.

APA Presidential Task Force on Evidence-Based Practice. (2006). Evidence-based practice in psychology. *American Psychologist*, 61(4), 271–285.

Aron, L. (1996). *A meeting of minds: Mutuality in psychoanalysis*. Hillsdale, NJ: The Analytic Press.

Aronson, M. (1956, January). Psychiatric management of disturbed behavior in a home for the aged. *Geriatrics*, 39–43.

Atkinson, J.M. (2007). *Advance directives in mental health: Theory, practice and ethics*. Philadelphia: Jessica Kingsley Publishers.

Avorn, J., Langer, E. (1982). Induced disability in nursing home patients: A controlled trial. *Journal of the American Geriatric Society*, 30, 397–400.

Banziger, G. & Roush, S. (1983). Nursing homes for the birds: A control-relevant intervention with bird feeders. *The Gerontologist*, 23(5), 527–531.

Barns, E.K., Sack, A., & Shore, H. (1973, Winter). Guidelines to treatment approaches: Modalities for use with the aged. *The Gerontologist*, 513–527.

Beck, C., Heacock, P., Mercer, S.O., Walls, R.C., Rapp, C.G., & Vogelpohl, T.S. (1997). Improving dressing behavior in cognitively impaired nursing home residents. *Nursing Research*, 46, 126–132.

Beck, C., Ortigara, A., Mercer, S.O., and Shue, V. (1999). Enabling and empowering certified nursing assistants for quality dementia care. *International Journal of Geriatric Psychiatry*, 14, 197–212.

Berlin, L.J., Cassidy, J., & Appleyard, K. (2008). The influence of early attachments on other relationships. In J. Cassidy & P.E. Shaver (Eds.), *Handbook of attachment* (2nd ed., pp. 333–347). New York: Gilford Press.

Borson, S., Reichman, W.E., Coyne, A.C., Rovner, B., Sakauye, K. (2000). Effectiveness of nursing home staff as managers of disruptive behavior: Perceptions of nursing directors. *American Journal of Geriatric Psychiatry*, 8(3), 251–253.

Bouklas, G. (1997). *Psychotherapy with the elderly: Becoming Methuselah's echo*. Northvale, NJ: Jason Aronson.

Brandtstadter, J., & Baltes-Gotz, B. (1990). Personal control over development and quality of life perspectives in adulthood. In P.B. Baltes & M.M. Baltes (Eds.), *Successful aging* (pp. 197–224). Cambridge, England: Cambridge University Press.

Brazil, K., Hasler, A., McAiney, C., Sturdy-Smith, C., Tettman, M. (2003). *Journal of Mental Health and Aging* 9(1), 35–42.

Burgio, L.D., Allen-Burge, R., Roth, D.L., Bourgeois, M.S., Dijkstra, K., & Gerstle, J. (2001). Come talk with me: Improving communication between nursing assistants and nursing home residents during care routines. *The Gerontologist*, 41(4), 449–460.

Burgio, L.D. & Bourgeois, M.S. (1992). Treating severe behavioral disorders in geriatric residential settings. *Behavioral Residential Treatment*, 7, 145–168.

Burgio, L.D., & Burgio, K.L. (1990). Institutional staff training and management. *The International Journal of Aging and Human Development*, 30(4), 287–302.

Burgio, L.D., & Burgio, K.L. (1986). Behavioral gerontology: Application of behavioral methods to problems of older adults. *Journal of Applied Behavior Analysis, 19,* 321–328.

Burgio, L.D., Jones, L.T., Butler, F., & Engel, B.T. (1988). The prevalence of geriatric behavior problems in an urban nursing home. *Gerontological Nursing, 14*(1), 31–34.

Burgio, L.D., & Stevens, A.B. (1998). Behavioral interventions and motivational systems in the nursing home. *Annual Review of Gerontology and Geriatrics, 18,* 284–320.

Burgio, L.D., Stevens, A., Burgio, K.L., Roth, D.L., Paul, P., & Gerstle, J. (2002). Teaching and maintaining behavior management skills in the nursing home. *The Gerontologist, 42*(4), 487–496.

Carr, L. Iacoboni, M., Dubeau, M., Mazziotta, J.C., & Lenzi, G.L. Neural mechanisms of empathy in humans: A relay from neural systems for imitation to limbic areas. *Proceedings of the National Academy of Sciences, 100*(9), 5497–5502.

Chafetz, P.K. (1996). Behavioral management of secondary symptoms of dementia. In R.L. Dippel & J.T. Hutton (Eds.), *Caring for the Alzheimer patient: A practical guide* (pp. 123–133). Amherst, NY: Prometheus Books.

Cohen-Mansfield, J., Marx, M.S., & Rosenthal, A.S. (1989). A description of agitation in the nursing home. *Journal of Gerontological Medical Science, 44,* 77–84.

Cohen-Mansfield, J., Marx, M.S., & Rosenthal, A.S. (1990). Screaming in nursing home residents. *Journal of the American Geriatric Society, 38,* 785–792.

Cohler, B.J. (1998). Psychoanalysis and the life course: Development and intervention. In I.H. Nordhus, G.R. VandenBos, S. Berg, & P. Fromholt (Eds.), *Clinical geropsychology* (pp. 79–108). Washington, DC: American Psychological Association.

Cohn, M.D., Smyer, M.A., & Horgas, A.L. (1994). *The ABCs of behavior change: Skills for working with behavior problems in nursing homes.* State College, PA: Ventura Publishing.

Colarusso, C.A., & Nemiroff, R.A. (1981). *Adult development.* New York: Plenum Press.

Dinkmeyer, D., McKay, G.D., McKay, J.L., & Dinkmeyer, D. Jr. (1998). *Parenting teens: Systematic training for effective parenting.* Circle Pines, MN: AGS Publishing.

Davidhizar, R. (2004). Listening—a nursing strategy to transcend culture. *Journal of Practical Nursing, 54*(2), 22–24.

Elbogen, E.B., Van Doren, R., Swanson, J.W., Swartz, M.S., Feron, J., Wagner, H.R., & Wilder, C. (2007). Effectively implementing psychiatric advance directives to promote self-determination of treatment among people with mental illness. *Psychology, Public Policy, and the Law, 13*(4): 10.1037/1076–8971.13.4.273.

Erikson, E.H. (1982). *The life cycle completed.* New York: W.W. Norton & Company.

Feil, N. (2012). *The Validation breakthrough: Simple techniques for communicating with people with Alzheimer's and other dementias* (3rd ed.). Baltimore: Health Professions Press.

Finkel, S.I. (1993). Diagnosis and treatment of delirium in the nursing home. In P.A. Szwabo & G.T. Grossberg (Eds.), *Problem behaviors in long-term care: Recognition, diagnosis, and treatment* (pp. 110–121). New York: Springer-Verlag.

Gerwood, J.B. (1993). Nondirective counseling interventions with schizophrenics. *Psychological Reports, 73,* 1147–1151.

Gallagher-Thompson, D., & Coon, D.W. (2007). Evidence-based treatments to reduce psychological distress in family caregivers of older adults. *Psychology and Aging, 22,* 37–51.

Gallagher-Thompson, D., Ossindale, C., & Thompson, L.W. (1999). *Coping with caregiving: A class for family caregivers*. Unpublished manuscript, Veterans Administration Palo Alto Healthcare System and Stanford University School of Medicine.

Gallese, V. (2003). The roots of empathy: The shared manifold hypothesis and the neural basis of intersubjectivity. *Psychopathology, 36*, 171–180.

Gallese, V. (2001). The shared manifold hypothesis: From mirror neurons to empathy. *Journal of Consciousness Studies, 8*(5–7), 33–50.

Gatz, M. (2000). Variations on depression in later life. In S.H. Qualls & N. Abeles (Eds.), *Psychology and the aging revolution: How we adapt to longer life* (pp. 239–254). Washington, DC: American Psychological Association.

Gubrium, J.F. (1997). *Living and dying at Murray Manor*. Charlottesville: The University of Virginia Press.

Gwyther, L.P. (1986, May). Treating behavior as a symptom of illness. *Provider*, 18–21.

Henderson, J.N. (1995). The culture of care in a nursing home: Effects of a medicalized model of long-term care. In J.N. Henderson & M.D. Vesperi (Eds.), *The culture of long-term care: Nursing home ethnography* (pp. 37–54). Westport, CT: Bergin & Garvey.

Jencks, S.F., & Clauser, S.B. (1991). Improving nursing home care through training and job redesign. *The Gerontologist, 32*(2), 327–333.

Jenike, M. (1988). Depression and other psychiatric disorders. In M.S. Albert & M.B. Moss (Eds.), *Geriatric neuropsychology* (pp. 115–144). New York: The Guilford Press.

Joiner, T.E. (2000). Depression: Current developments and controversies. In S.H. Qualls & N. Abeles (Eds.), *Psychology and the aging revolution: How we adapt to longer life* (pp. 223–237). Washington, DC: American Psychological Association.

Kahneman, D. (2011). *Thinking fast and slow*. New York: Farrar, Straus and Giroux.

Karon, B.P., & VanderBos, G.R. (1998). Schizophrenia and psychosis in elderly populations. In I.H. Nordhus, G.R. VandenBos, S. Berg, & P. Fromholt (Eds.), *Clinical geropsychology* (pp. 219–227). Washington, DC: American Psychological Association.

Kasl-Godley, J.E., Gatz, M., & Fiske, A. (1998). Depression and depressive symptoms in old age. In I.H. Nordhus, G.R. VandenBos, S. Berg, & P. Fromholt (Eds.), *Clinical geropsychology* (pp. 211–217). Washington, DC: American Psychological Association.

Keane, B., & Dixon, C. (2001). *Caring for people with behavior problems: A basic, practical text for nurses, health workers and others who are learning to manage difficult behaviors*. Melbourne, Australia: Ausmed Publications.

Krantz D.S., & Schulz, P.R. (1980). Personal control and health: Some applications to crises of middle and old age. *Advances in Environmental Psychology, 2*, 23–57.

Kübler-Ross, E. (1969). *On death and dying: What the dying have to teach doctors, nurses, clergy, and their own families*. New York: Collier Books.

Lach, H.W. (1993). Use of physical restraints and options. In P.A. Szwabo & G.T. Grossberg (Eds.), *Problem behaviors in long-term care: Recognition, diagnosis, and treatment* (pp. 176–187). New York: Springer-Verlag.

Lazarus, R.S. (1998). Coping with aging: Individuality as a key to understanding. In I.H. Nordhus, G.R. VandenBos, S. Berg, & P. Fromholt (Eds.), *Clinical geropsychology* (pp. 109–127). Washington, DC: American Psychological Association.

Le Blanc, L.A., Raetz, P., B., & Feliciano, L. (2011). Behavioral gerontology. In W.W. Fisher, C.C. Piazza, & H.S. Roane (Eds.), *Handbook of applied behavioral analysis* (pp. 472–486). New York: Guilford Press.

Lewinsohn, P.M., Antonuccio, D.O., Brechenridge, J.S., & Teri, L. (1984). *The coping with depression course*. Eugene, OR: Castalia Publishing Company.

Lewinsohn, P.M., Muñoz, R.F., Youngren, M.A., & Zeiss, A.M. (1986). *Control your depression: Reducing depression through learning self-control techniques, relaxation training, pleasant activities, social skills, constructed thinking, planning ahead, and more*. New York: Fireside.

Lipson, S. (1994). The restraint-free approach to behavior problems in the nursing home. *Maryland Medical Journal, 43*(2), 155–157.

Livingston, G., Johnston, K., Katona, C., Paton, J., & Lyketsos, C.G. (2005). Systematic review of psychological approaches to the management of neuropsychiatric symptoms of dementia. *American Journal of Psychiatry, 162*(11), 1996–2021.

Logsdon, R.G., McCurry, S.M., & Teri, L. (2007). Evidence-based psychological treatments for disruptive behaviors in individuals with dementia. *Psychology and Aging, 22*(1), 28–36.

Lomranz, J. (1991). Mental health in homes for the aged and the clinical psychology of aging: Implementation of a model service. *Clinical Gerontologist, 10*(3), 47–72.

Long, S.W. (2007). A relational perspective on working with dying patients in a nursing home setting. In B. Willock, L.C. Bohm, & R.C. Curtis (Eds.), *On deaths and endings: psychoanalysists' reflections on finality, transformations and new beginnings* (pp. 237–246). New York: Routledge.

Luborsky, L., & Luborsky, E. (2006). *Research and psychotherapy*. New York: Jason Aronson.

Luskin, F. (2002). *Forgive for good: A proven prescription for health and happiness*. San Francisco: HarperCollins.

Mahoney, E.K., Volicer, L., & Hurley, A.C. (2000). *Management of challenging behaviors in dementia*. Baltimore: Health Professions Press.

Main, M., Kaplan, N., & Cassidy, J. (1985). Security in infancy, childhood, and adulthood: A move to the level of representation. *Applied Psychology, 84*, 754–775.

Mallinckrodt, B. (2010). The psychotherapy relationship as attachment: Evidence and implications. *Journal of Social and Personal Relations, 27*(2), 262–270.

McCabe, M.P., Davison, T.E., & George, K. (2007). Effectiveness of staff training programs for behavioral problems among older people with dementia. *Aging and Mental Health, 11*(5), 505–519.

McCallion, P., Toseland, R.W., Lacey, D., & Banks, S. (1999). Educating nursing assistants to communicate more effectively with nursing home residents with dementia. *The Gerontologist, 39*, 546–558.

McCarthy, J.F., Blow, F.C., & Kales, H.C. (2004). Disruptive behaviors in Veterans Affairs nursing home residents: How different are residents with serious mental illness? *American Geriatrics Society, 52*, 2031–2038.

McCleary, R.W. (1992). *Conversing with uncertainty: Practicing psychotherapy in a hospital setting*. Hillsdale, NJ: The Analytic Press.

Meyers, B.S., & Cahenzi, C.T. (1993). Psychotropics in the extended care facility. In P.A. Szwabo & G.T. Grossberg (Eds.), *Problem behaviors in long-term care: Recognition, diagnosis, and treatment* (pp. 81–93). New York: Springer-Verlag.

Mineyama, S., Tsutsumi, A., Takao, S., Nishiuchi, K., & Kawakami, N. (2007). Supervisors' attitudes and skills for active listening with regard to working conditions and psychological distress reactions among subordinate workers. *Journal of Occupational Health, 49*(2), 81–87.

Mitchell, S.A., & Black, M.J. (1995). *Freud and beyond: A history of modern psychoanalytic thought*. New York: Basic Books.

Meeks, S., Looney, S.W., Van Haitsman, K., Teri, L. (2008). BE-ACTIV: A staff-assisted behavioral intervention for depression in nursing homes. *The Gerontologist*, 48(1), 105–114.

Morley, J.E., & Miller, D.K. (1993). Behavioral concomitants of common medical disorders. In P.A. Szwabo & G.T. Grossberg (Eds.), *Problem behaviors in long-term care: Recognition, diagnosis, and treatment* (pp. 97–109). New York: Springer-Verlag.

Nelson, J. (1995, May). The influence of environmental factors in incidents of disruptive behavior. *Journal of Gerontological Nursing*, 19–24.

Norcross, J.C., Beutler, L.E., & Levant, R.F. (Eds.) (2006). *Evidence-based practices in mental health*. Washington, DC: American Psychological Association.

Norcross, J.C., & Knight, B.G. (2000). Psychotherapy and aging in the 21st century: Integrative themes. In S.H. Qualls & N. Abeles (Eds.), *Psychology and the aging revolution: How we adapt to longer life* (pp. 259–286). Washington, DC: American Psychological Association.

Pinkston, E., & Linsk, N.L. (1984). *Care of the elderly: A family approach*. New York: Pergamon Press.

Ray, W.A., Taylor, J.A., Lichtenstein, M.J., Meador, K.G., Stovdemire, A., Lipton, B., & Blazer, D. (1991). Managing behavior problems in nursing home residents. *Contemporary Management in Internal Medicine*, 1, 71–112.

Ray, W.A., Taylor, J.A., Meador, K.G., Lichtenstein, M.J., Griffin, M.R., Fought, R., Adams, M.L., & Blazer, D.G. (1993). Reducing antipsychotic drug use in nursing homes: A controlled trial of provider education. *Archives of Internal Medicine*, 153, 713–721.

Rogers, J.C., Holm, M.B., Burgio, L.D., Granieri, E., Hsu, C., Hardin, M., & McDowell, B.J. (1999). Improving morning care routines of nursing home residents with dementia. *Journal of the American Geriatrics Society*, 47, 1049–1057.

Romeis, J.C. (1993). Problem behaviors among younger adult nursing home residents. In P.A. Szwabo & G.T. Grossberg (Eds.), *Problem behaviors in long-term care: Recognition, diagnosis, and treatment* (pp. 21–31). New York: Springer-Verlag.

Rosowsky, E., Casciani, J.M., Arnold, M. (Eds.) (2009). *Geropsychology and Long-Term Care*. New York: Springer.

Rovner, B.W., Lucas-Blaustein, J., Folstein, M.F., & Smith, S.W. (1990). Stability over one year in patients admitted to a nursing home dementia unit. *International Journal of Geriatric Psychiatry*, 5, 77–82.

Ryan, R.M., & LaGuardia, J.G. (2000). What is being optimized?: Self-determination theory and basic psychological needs. In S.H. Qualls & N. Abeles (Eds.), *Psychology and the aging revolution: How we adapt to longer life* (pp. 145–172). Washington, DC: American Psychological Association.

Schulz, P.R. (1976). Effect of control and predictability on the psychological well-being of the institutionalized aged. *Journal of Personality and Social Psychology*, 33, 563–573.

Scogin, F.R. (1998). Anxiety in old age. In I.H. Nordhus, G.R. VandenBos, S. Berg, & P. Fromholt (Eds.), *Clinical geropsychology* (pp. 205–209). Washington, DC: American Psychological Association.

Sky, A.J., & Grossberg, G.T., (1993). Aggressive behaviors and chemical restraints. In P.A. Szwabo & G.T. Grossberg (Eds.), *Problem behaviors in long-term care: Recognition, diagnosis, and treatment* (pp. 188–200). New York: Springer-Verlag.

Slochower, J.A. (1996). *Holding and psychoanalysis: A relational perspective*. Hillsdale, NJ: The Analytic Press. Smyer, M.A., Brannon, D., & Cohn, M. (1992). Improving nursing home care through training and job redesign. *The Gerontologist*, 32(2), 327–333.

Smyer, M.A., & Downs, M.G. (1995). Psychopharmacology: An essential element in educating clinical psychologists for working with older adults. In B.G. Knight, L. Teri, P. Wohlford, & J. Santos (Eds.), *Mental health services for older adults: Implications for training and practice in geropsychology* (pp. 73–83). Washington, DC: American Psychological Association.

Snowdon, J. (1993). Mental health in nursing homes: Perspectives on the use of medications. *Drugs and Aging*, 3(2), 122–130.

Solomon, K. (1993). Behavioral and psychotherapeutic interventions with residents in long-term care institutions. In P.A. Szwabo & G.T. Grossberg (Eds.), *Problem behaviors in long-term care: Recognition, diagnosis, and treatment* (pp. 147–162). New York: Springer-Verlag.

Sorensen, L., Foldspang, A., Gulmann, N.C., & Munk-Jorgensen, P. (2001). Determinants for the use of psychotropics among nursing home residents. *International Journal of Geriatric Psychiatry*, 16, 147–154.

Spayd, S.C., & Smyer, M.A. (1996). Psychological interventions in nursing homes. In S.H. Zarit & B.G. Knight (Eds.), *A guide to psychotherapy and aging* (pp. 241–268). Washington, DC: American Psychological Association.

Stevens, A.B., Burgio, L.D., Bailey, E., Burgio, K.L., Paul, P., Capilouto, E., Nicovich, P., & Hale, G. (1998). Teaching and maintaining behavior management skills with nursing assistants in a nursing home. *The Gerontologist*, 38(3), 379–384.

Streim, J.E., & Katz, I.R. (1994). Federal regulations and the care of patients with dementia in the nursing home. *Medical Clinics of North America*, 78(4), 895–909.

Szwabo, P.A., & Boesch, K.R. (1993). Impact of personality and personality disorders in the elderly. In P.A. Szwabo & G.T. Grossberg (Eds.), *Problem behaviors in long-term care: Recognition, diagnosis, and treatment* (pp. 59–69). New York: Springer-Verlag.

Taylor, R.L. (1990). *Distinguishing psychological from organic disorders: Screening for psychological masquerade*. New York: Springer-Verlag.

Teri, L. (1994). Behavioral treatment of depression in patients with dementia. *Alzheimer's Disease and Associated Disorders*, 8, 66–74.

Teri, L. (1990). Managing and understanding behavior problems in Alzheimer's and related disorders. (Training program with videotapes and written manual.) Seattle: University of Washington.

Teri, L. (1992). Non-pharmacological approaches to management of patient behavior: A focus on behavioral interventions for depression in dementia. In G. Gutman (Ed.), *Shelter and care of persons with dementia* (pp. 101–113). Vancouver, British Columbia, Canada: Simon Fraser University, The Gerontology Research Centre.

Teri, L., Huda, P., Gibbons, L., Young, H., van Leynseele, J. (2005). STAR: a dementia specific training program for staff in assisted living residences. *The Gerontologist*, 45(5), 686–693.

Teri, L., Rabins, P., Whitehouse, P., Berg, L. Reisperg, B. Sunderland, T., Eichelman, B., & Pheps, C. (1992). Management of behavior disturbance in Alzheimer disease: Current knowledge and future directions. *Alzheimer Disease and Associated Disorders*, 6(2), 77–88.

Teri, L., Mckenzie, G.L., Pike, K.C., Foran, C.J., Beck, C., Paun, O., & LaFazia, D. (2009). *American Journal of Geriatric Psychiatry*, 18(6), 502–509.

Teri, L., & Umoto, J.M. (1991). Reducing excess disability in dementia patients: Training caregivers to manage patient depression. *Clinical Gerontologist*, 10(4), 49–63.

Thomasma, M., Yeaworth, R., & McCabe, B. (1990). Moving day: Relocation and anxiety in institutional elderly. *Journal of Gerontological Nursing*, 16, 18–24.

Veterans Health Administration's Employee Education System. (2001). *Prevention and management of disruptive behavior*. Washington, DC: Veteran's Administration Office of Occupational Safety and Health.

Wachtel, P.L. (1997). *Psychoanalysis, behavior therapy, and the relational world*. Washington, DC: American Psychological Association.

Wachtel, P.L. (2008). *Relational Theory and the Practice of Psychotherapy*. New York: The Guilford Press.

Wachtel, P.L. (2011). *Therapeutic communication: Knowing what to say when*. New York: The Guilford Press.

Weiner, M.F., Tractenberg, R.E., Sano, M., Logsdon, R., Teri, L., Galasko, D., Gamst, R.T., & Thal, L.J. (2002). No long-term effect of behavioral treatment on psychotropic drug use for agitation in Alzheimer's disease patients. *Journal of Geriatric Psychiatry and Neurology*, 15, 95–98.

Westen, D. (1999). The scientific status of unconscious processes: Is Freud really dead? *Journal of the American Psychoanalytic Association*, 47, 1061–1106.

Whitbourne, S.K. (1998). Physical changes in the aging individual: Clinical implications. In I.H. Nordhus, G.R. VandenBos, S. Berg, & P. Fromholt (Eds.), *Clinical geropsychology* (pp. 79–108). Washington, DC: American Psychological Association.

Zarit, S.H. (1996). Ethical considerations in the treatment of older adults. In S.H. Zarit & B.G. Knight (Eds.), *A guide to psychotherapy and aging* (pp. 269–284). Washington, DC: American Psychological Association.

Zarit, S.H., Dolan, M.M., & Leitsch, S.A. (1998). Interventions in nursing homes and alternate living settings. In I.H. Nordhus, G.R. VandenBos, S. Berg, & P. Fromholt (Eds.), *Clinical geropsychology* (pp. 329–343). Washington, DC: American Psychological Association.

Zarit, S.H. & Zarit, J.M. (2007). *Mental disorders in older adults*. New York: the Guilford Press.

The following forms are also available for *free* download at www.healthpropress. com/caring-downloadable-resources (use password m2f37rg).

Blank Forms

Top 10 Pleasant Events List

Pleasant Events Tracking Form

New Top 10 Pleasant Events List

ABCs of Behavior Observation Form

ABCs of Thinking and Feeling Form

Basic Psychological Skills Evaluation Form

Advance Directive: Mental Health/Behavioral Health/Stress Management

Top 10 Pleasant Events List

1. _____

2. _____

3. _____

4. _____

5. _____

6. _____

7. _____

8. _____

9. _____

10. _____

List 10 small, pleasant activities you like to do. Make sure that the activities are realistic, "do-able" things such as taking a short walk, talking with a friend, sitting alone quietly, holding hands with a loved one, or watching a favorite television program.

Include activities that you do not already do often. Rank the items, placing the one that is most important to you at the top of the list.

Pleasant Events Tracking Form

	Day & Date	Day & Date	Day & Date	Day & Date	Day & Date	Day & Date	Day & Date
Pleasant Events							
1							
2							
3							
4							
5							
6							
7							
8							
9							
10							
Totals for each day							

List your top 10 pleasant events in the lefthand column. Record the day and date you start tracking at the top of the next column. Record the day and date of the following 6 days over the remaining columns.

In the column below each day and date, place a check mark in the appropriate box when one of your pleasant activities has occurred. Even if you experience the same event numerous times in one day, place only one check mark in the box. For example, if one of your pleasant events is reading the newspaper, only check the corresponding activity and date box one time, even if you sit down to read the paper four times that day.

At the end of each day, count the number of check marks in that day's column. Record the number of check marks for that day in the box at the bottom of the column.

Your goal may be to have more of your top 10 pleasant events each day than recorded on the list.

New Top 10 Pleasant Events List

1. _____

2. _____

3. _____

4. _____

5. _____

6. _____

7. _____

8. _____

9. _____

10. _____

After a week of tracking your top 10 pleasant events, use this form to update your list. Replace anything from the previous list that you were not able to do. Or leave some of these items on the list for one more week if you think that you will be more able to do them now.

Use a copy of this form each week. Remove items from earlier Top 10 Lists that were unrealistic. Remove other activities that have become routine—that is, the ones that you now experience very often. Substitute do-able pleasant activities that you do not already do often. Rank the items, beginning with the one that you value most. Use the Pleasant Events Tracking Form to tally how many of your new Top 10 pleasant events you have each week.

ABCs of Behavior Observation Form

Date:	Time:	
A **Antecedent**	**B** **Behavior**	**C** **Consequence**

Date:	Time:	
A **Antecedent**	**B** **Behavior**	**C** **Consequence**

Date:	Time:	
A **Antecedent**	**B** **Behavior**	**C** **Consequence**

ABCs of Thinking and Feeling Form

Date:			
A **Activating Event**	**B** **Beliefs/Thoughts**	**C** **Emotional** **Consequences**	**D** **Disputing** **Beliefs/Thoughts**

Basic Psychological Skills Evaluation Form

Staff member: _____

Supervisor: _____ Date: _____

Instructions for the supervisor: This chart delineates 14 skills for evaluation. The first 12 skills relate to the staff member's work with care recipients and should be evaluated according to his or her application with those who engage in challenging behavior and routinely with all care recipients. (For your reference, descriptions of all 14 skill areas follow the chart.) Use these keys for indicating the staff member's ability in each area:

Performance ratings: E = Excellent
                                  G = Good
                                  S = Satisfactory
                                  I = Improving/Needs Improvement

Assessment based on: R = Staff member's report
                                  D = Documentation
                                  O = Observation by supervisor

Skills assessed	Assessment based on (Circle all that apply)				Assessment based on (Circle all that apply)		
1. Uses listening skills	E	G	S	I	R	D	O
2. Allows care recipients to make choices	E	G	S	I	R	D	O
3. Determines triggers and reinforcers of difficult behavior	E	G	S	I	R	D	O
4. Uses social reinforcers to encourage positive behaviors	E	G	S	I	R	D	O
5. Encourages care recipients to be actively involved in problem solving (as much as residents are able)	E	G	S	I	R	D	O
6. Effectively addresses attention-seeking behavior that is disruptive	E	G	S	I	R	D	O
7. Responds well to angry, hostile, or agitated behavior	E	G	S	I	R	D	O
8. Avoids negative approaches to difficult behaviors	E	G	S	I	R	D	O
9. Sets realistic goals for addressing difficult behaviors	E	G	S	I	R	D	O

10. Considers how difficult behaviors may be signs of psychological distress	E	G	S	I	R	D	O
11. Consults with others when having difficulty addressing a problem behavior	E	G	S	I	R	D	O
12. Spends at least 2–5 daily minutes visiting with each assigned or scheduled care recipient	E	G	S	I	R	D	O
13. Recognizes the importance of managing his or her own stress	E	G	S	I	R	D	O
14. Identifies potentially helpful methods of coping with stress that affects work performance	E	G	S	I	R	D	O

Comments:

Descriptions of the 14 Basic Psychological Skills

1. Uses listening skills: The staff member shows signs of paying attention, such as stopping whatever he or she is doing, making eye contact, nodding his or her head, and so forth. He or she accepts and names residents' feelings and accurately restates to care recipients what they say.

2. Allows care recipients to make choices: The staff member uses open-ended questions (e.g., "When would you like to go to bed?") with those who are interested in and able to make decisions. He or she uses limited-choice questions (e.g., "I can help you now or after your television program. Which would you prefer?") with those who are interested in and able to make decisions and with those who have difficulty with open-ended questions because of confusion, bad moods, or low motivation. The staff member uses open-ended questions more often than limited-choice questions with care recipients who are comfortable with and able to respond to them. He or she gives clear, step-by-step explanations to person's who are very confused or do not respond to questions. The staff member recognizes resistance or agitation at such times as possible indications of the person's choice to reject what is being done. The staff member respects this choice as long as it does not pose risks to the well-being and safety of the individual or others.

3. Determines triggers and reinforcers of difficult behavior: The staff member examines episodes of difficult behavior to understand what triggers the difficult behavior and if the behavior continues or worsens, what reinforces it.

4. Uses social reinforcers to encourage positive behaviors: The staff member uses praise, compliments, and acknowledgement of care recipients' efforts and positive or improved behaviors. He or she makes at least four positive comments for every one comment on a negative behavior.

5. Encourages care recipients to be actively involved in problem solving (as much as residents are able): The staff member listens to their points of view regarding problems. He or she asks them what has usually resolved these or similar problems in the past, then works with them to select possible solutions.

6. Effectively addresses attention-seeking behavior that is disruptive: The staff member works to meet care recipients' needs for attention and works toward gradual improvement in their ability to tolerate longer periods of independence.

7. Responds well to angry, hostile, or agitated behavior: The staff member is alert to signs that the care recipient is becoming agitated (e.g., shouting demands, making threats). He or she gives them space at such times. The staff member may describe limited choices for agitated individuals such as, "If you speak more calmly to me, I'll try to help you" or "If you shout at me again, I'll leave you on your own for about 15 minutes." (The staff member only does the latter if leaving does not put anyone at immediate risk of harm.) The staff member avoids getting defensive or counteraggressive.

8. Avoids negative approaches to difficult behaviors: The staff member avoids all of the following: nagging; arguing; making repeated demands; making threats; retaliating; withholding privileges; scolding; reprimanding; punishing; insisting that things are not the way care recipients see them; laughing at them; making them the butt of jokes; engaging in power struggles; and showing annoyance, frustration, or anger. He or she also avoids labeling difficult or agitated behavior as "unpredictable" or "unprovoked" and instead tries to identify and address triggers and reinforcers. The staff member acts in ways that model positive reactions to difficult circumstances and feelings.

9. Sets realistic goals for addressing difficult behaviors: The staff member realizes that behavior change is often gradual. He or she remembers that improvement is evident when difficult behaviors lessen in frequency or intensity or when behavioral episodes shorten. He or she recognizes that these changes can take longer with those with histories of long-established behavior patterns. He or she avoids overgeneralizing (e.g., seeing someone who engages in a challenging behavior as *always* behaving in difficult ways) and "catastrophizing" (e.g., seeing unpleasant, unfortunate behavior as *completely* terrible, horrible, or dangerous).

10. Considers how difficult behaviors may be signs of psychological distress: The staff member examines whether problem behaviors are motivated by unmet needs (e.g., the need for attention or for a sense of control, power, or effectiveness). He or she helps care recipients meet those needs.

11. Consults with others when having difficulty addressing a problem behavior: The staff member uses his or her supervisor and other staff members as resources. He or or she talks to and watches others who have more success in working with problem behaviors or with a particular care recipient. The staff member uses this information to find new ways of addressing persistent problems.

12. Spends at least 2–5 minutes daily visiting with each assigned or scheduled care recipient: The staff member spends time with care recipients each day. If chatting with them, he or she emphasizes active listening. During this time, the staff member engages in activities that care recipients initiate or prefer (e.g., watching television, walking, people watching, sitting in the sun, listening to music, discussing news).

13. Recognizes the importance of managing his or her own stress: The staff member recognizes that his or her ability to manage stress affects how well he or she uses basic skills. He or she sees lack of improvement in care recipients' problem behaviors as a possible sign that his or her stress level is interfering with effective use of basic skills.

14. Identifies potentially helpful methods of coping with stress that affects work performance: The staff member can state how stress may be better managed by strategies such as engaging in team work, being open to different approaches to problems, and being open to different ways of thinking about problems that have considerable support in clinical and research literature.

Advance Directive:
Mental Health/Behavioral Health/Stress Management

If you have a significant health problem, important changes in your life, notable challenges you face, or a mental illness, you can experience stress. Stress is sometimes called being under pressure or feeling tense, jumpy, blue, down in the dumps, irritable, or grumpy. It is often experienced as physical problems, such as headaches, fatigue, or upset stomach. Stress can have a negative effect on your emotions, your activities, and your ability to get along with others. Significant stress can affect how well you understand information, think, or make decisions. Strong or persistent stress can have a negative impact on mental health or general health. Preventing or reducing the stress you feel can be an important part of your overall healthcare.

Think about your experience with stress. If you recognize that it can negatively affect your emotions and how you behave, or if you know that stress worsens your mental or general health, you may want your healthcare providers and loved ones to know what they can do to help you.

You can use this form to let them know:
- the signs that you are feeling too stressed
- what they can do to help

This form is to be completed when you are not too ill or too stressed to express your wishes clearly. It is for you to fill out when you are able to think clearly enough to make informed decisions about what you would like done in response to signs that you are too stressed.

Initials:_____   Date last updated_____

Page_____

Part 1A. Statement of my intentions

I _____, being of sound mind, voluntarily provide the following healthcare instructions. I provide these instructions now in case, at some time in the future, I am unable to clearly express my wishes or am unable to make informed decisions due to illness or due to my experience of circumstances that led to a level of stress that interferes with my thinking clearly enough to make informed decisions about my care.

In any stress management or mental health situation that is not covered by this document, I designate _____ as my proxy to make decisions regarding my care if I am unable to think clearly enough to make informed decisions about my care or if I am unable to express my decisions.

Part 1B. Statement of my intentions

(To be completed by the designated healthcare proxy, or other appropriately designated person, if a mental health, behavioral health, or stress management advance directive has not been documented for _____ prior to the time he/she was unable to think clearly enough to make informed decisions or was unable to express them.)

As the healthcare proxy (or other appropriately designated person) for_____,
I _____ being of sound mind, voluntarily provide the following healthcare instructions. I provide these instructions now in case, at some time in the future, I am unable to express them or am unable to make informed decisions due to illness or due to my experience of circumstances which led to a level of stress that interferes with my thinking clearly.

Statements or requests made in the remainder of this document are often made in the first person (for example, "Please recognize that I am experiencing stress"). Although I am completing this form, these statements or requests are intended to be understood as those of _____ (name of care recipient).

Initials:_____   Date last updated_____

Page_____

Part 2. Statement of my wishes

1. Please recognize the signs that I am experiencing stress.

The checked items below are signs that I am stressed and that the stress may be worsening.

Signs of Stress

Feelings	Thinking	Behavior	Interactions with Others
I often or strongly express that I feel:	I often or strongly say:	I often or strongly:	I often or strongly:
__Unhappy, sad, or down	__ Any of the following: I am not worth much/No one cares	__Do any of the following: Very little/ Cry/Sleep too much or too little/Eat too much or too little	__Withdraw and isolate myself
__Anxiety or fear	__Any of the following: I am worried, frightened, or scared/I am not safe/Something bad is going to happen/ What I need is withheld/I am going to be harmed or retaliated against	__Do any of the following: Call for someone to come to me or for help/ Try not to be alone/ Move restlessly/ Have trouble concentrating	__Try to be with others or have them stay with me
__Frustration, irritation, or anger	__Any of the following: I am dissatisfied/I should be able to do what I cannot do/ Others should do what they have not done/Others have to stop doing what they are doing/ Others disrespect me or my rights/ There is too much of what I do not like happening and it must stop	__Do any of the following: Talk loudly/Use strong language/argue, demand, or disagree loudly/Shout/ Scream	__Any of the following: I sternly express dissatisfaction toward others/I demand or insist that others do, or stop doing, something/I strongly state that there will be negative consequences if what I believe must be done is not done/I firmly state to others my negative evaluations of them/I can be hard to get along with

Initials:_____   Date last updated_____

Page_____

Other signs that I am stressed and that my stress may be worsening are:

2. Protective Factors

The following checked items may help me avoid significant levels of stress when they are part of my routine treatment. These are also factors that can help reduce my stress once it has reached a high level. Detailed descriptions of these Essentials of Care are on the three pages immediately following the checklist.

Initials:_____   Date last updated_____

Page_____

Essentials of Care*

Check all that apply.

1___ Listening
2___ Allowing choices
3___ Letting me know that you notice improvements in what I do, even small ones
4___ Letting me know you see my positive efforts
5___ Finding what triggers my stressed behavior, including when interacting with others
6___ Finding what reinforces my stressed behavior, including when interacting with others
7___ Supporting my positive efforts at coping with stress Learning about how I effectively coped in the past
8___ Helping by changing the factors external to me that trigger or reinforce my stressed behavior
9___ Recognizing and responding to my need for attention
10___ Avoiding arguing, making repeated demands, or scolding
11___ Avoiding labeling my stressed or challenging behavior as "unpredictable" or "unprovoked" (see items 7 and 8)
12___ Giving me space and time to calm down
13___ Recognizing signs of your own stress when dealing with mine Taking care of yourself is important
14___ If my behavior remains very stressed or challenging, or becomes more so, consulting with others who have found effective ways of dealing with similar situations

*See the following three pages for detailed descriptions of each of these Essentials of Care.

Initials:_____   Date last updated_____

Page_____

Detailed Description of the Essentials of Care

1. Being listened to. Having someone actively listen can be very helpful. This involves the person who is listening stopping whatever else he or she is doing and showing that he or she hears and understands what I am saying. Signs that he or she is doing this include eye contact and accurately restating what I am trying to say and how I feel.

2. Being allowed to make choices. This can be done, for example, with questions such as:

"When would you like to go to bed?"
"I can help you now or after your television program. Which would you prefer?

If I am ever very confused, forgetful, or stressed, making choices may be too difficult. It could trigger more stress. At these times, clear step-by-step explanations of what others are helping me with can be helpful.

Please, at such times, recognize that resistance or agitation on my part may be indications of my choice that what is being done stop. When this happens, please respect this choice, as long as doing so does not put anyone at immediate risk of significant harm.

3 and 4. Having improvements in what I do, even small improvements, and positive things I do in general, be noticed. Having others let me know when they see things I do that are positive efforts. It is encouraging when others acknowledge my positive efforts and improvements. Sometimes it helps me to know that I am on the right track and that continuing my efforts could be fruitful.

5 and 6. Having others see what triggers my stressed behavior, including the triggers during interactions with others. Having others see what reinforces my stressed behavior, including during interactions with others. Stress-related behaviors, like all behaviors, are triggered by something. When they continue or get stronger, something is reinforcing them. Triggers and reinforcers can include factors such as illness, pain, medications, discomfort, or unpleasant events. Often the most important sources of triggers and reinforcers of positive behaviors are interactions with other people. The same is true of stress-related or challenging behavior. Even when someone has the best intentions, when the other person in an interaction becomes increasingly stressed, some aspect of the interaction is likely to be triggering and reinforcing that stress.

7. Having others support my positive efforts at coping with stress. Having others understand how my stress has successfully been coped with in the past. It is helpful when others listen to my point of view regarding signs that I am stressed and what can be done about it. I have been stressed before and have had some success in dealing with it. Sometimes the efforts I have made that have worked well for me in the past I, or others, can still make.

Initials:_____   Date last updated_____

Page_____

8. Having others help by changing the external factors that trigger or reinforce my stressed behavior, including the triggers and reinforces during interactions with others. Unpleasant events, an overly stimulating (or under stimulating) environment, and the demands of others are examples of triggers and reinforcers of stress. Other triggers and reinforcers are likely to be such factors as my not feeling understood (or not listened to well), not having been allowed to make routine choices, having my choices regularly given little priority, having others respond only to (or mostly to) the negatives about me or the things I do, or being ignored. Some of the most important triggers or reinforcers for how I feel are often how my interactions go with other people.

9. Having my need to be paid attention to recognized and responded to. Being positively responded to by others can help prevent or reduce my stress. This could mean such things as simply being greeted or being given assistance that I've requested in a timely way. It could mean having regular visits from others (including staff) with whom I have good relationships. Such visits would not be to administer other medical/nursing assistance. These visits could be for as little as 2 to 5 minutes and would involve chatting or even sitting quietly together.

10. Having others avoid arguing with me, making repeated demands, or scolding me. Often arguing, making demands, and scolding add to my stress and make stress-related behaviors more likely.

11. Having others avoid labeling my stressed or challenging behavior "unpredictable" or "unprovoked" (see items 5 through 7). Instead of labeling signs that I am stressed as unpredictable or unprovoked, please understand that when a behavior seems that way, it can be understood better. Behaviors happen for reasons. The reasons may not be obvious, but when they are not, please carefully assess the circumstances in which they happen. Understanding what triggers and reinforces stress or stress-related behavior is important for reducing the stress and the related behavior.

12. Being given space and time to calm down. If I am being very hard to get along with, please give me some time and space. Often, after a short period of time (sometimes as little as 15 to 20 minutes) I behave in a less stressed way. At times like these you might say something such as, "I'd like to help you, but it is difficult for me to do that while you are yelling at me. Should I stay now and help you, or should I come back in about 15 minutes." Or even, "If we have more trouble getting along right now, I'll leave you on your own for about 15 minutes." I understand that you would not be able to leave me if doing so puts anyone, including me, at immediate, significant risk of harm.

Initials:_____   Date last updated_____

Page_____

13. Having others recognize signs of their own stress when dealing with mine. Having others take care of their own stress because it is important that they take good care of themselves. Stress in relationships can be contagious. I will do my best to deal with my stress, including with the help of others. When I am too stressed or ill, I know that my stress can be challenging for others. Please, do your best to take care of yourself, too, including with the help of others.

14. If my behavior remains very stressed or challenging or becomes more so, consult with others who have found effective ways of dealing with similar situations. Talk with and watch others who have had success in interacting with me or with other people who are stressed or showing signs of stress.

Initials:_____   Date last updated_____

Page_____

3. Treatment Preferences

If my level of stress and stress-related behaviors call for a formal treatment plan, or if they rise to the level of a diagnosable mental illness, I wish (check all that apply):

_____that the initial treatment plan not include medication.

_____that the initial treatment plan and subsequent treatment plans state:

- how triggers and reinforcers of the stress that may contribute to my symptoms and stress-related behaviors or mental illness will be identified (see Essentials of Care).
- how identified triggers and reinforcers will be modified to reduce the stress (see Essentials of Care).

_____that I receive psychological therapy or counseling at a frequency and duration that is appropriate for my needs

_____that any medication treatment I agree to receive for mental health, behavioral health, or stress management be used in the following manner:

- there will be appropriate indications for use
- there will be a specific and documented goal for the use of the medication
- there will be ongoing monitoring to evaluate the medication's effectiveness in reaching the goal and to identify any adverse effects from the medication
- medication will only be used as long as needed and at the lowest dose necessary for reaching the goal

4. Medication Instructions

I agree to receive the following medication(s) (if indicated), because they have helped me in the past:

Initials:_____   Date last updated_____

Page_____

If reasonable alternatives exist, I would like to avoid the following medications. (Identify the reasons for your preferences. For example, bad side effects or concern about long-term side effects or whether the medication did not work when your symptoms were worse.)

I do not agree to the following medication(s).

I understand that medications may cause side effects. However, if there are reasonable alternatives, I especially would like to avoid the following bad side effects (check up to four):

_____Unusual movements of my mouth or other areas

_____Numbness (loss of sensation)

_____Motor restlessness (not being able to sit still or stand without moving around)

_____Seizures (During a seizure, your body twitches or shakes for a brief period of time. You cannot control your body and you usually become unconscious.)

_____Stiffness in my muscles or body, so that I cannot smoothly or normally move my arms, legs, or body

_____Tremors (An example of a tremor is when your hands shake or vibrate very fast and you cannot control it.)

_____Nausea or vomiting (feeling sick to your stomach or throwing up)

_____Gaining weight

_____Losing weight

_____Diabetes (Diabetes is a condition that causes problems in maintaining your normal blood sugar and is sometimes called the "sugar disease.")

_____Problems with my sexual functioning

_____Addiction or dependence to the medication(s)

_____Other:

Initials:_____   Date last updated_____

Page_____

5. Entering a Mental Health Facility/Unit

If I need to be hospitalized, or transferred to a specialty unit, for mental health problems, there will be a plan specifying the goal of the inpatient treatment and discharge once the goal is reached.

_____ Yes

_____ No

I agree to admission to the following hospitals or units:

I do not agree to admission to the following hospitals or units:

6. Other Information and Instructions

In case of a mental health crisis, the crisis unit or hospital should know that the following might help me get my mental health symptoms under control:

Initials:_____   Date last updated_____

Page_____

The staff should know that the following might help me relax and be less agitated, and also might lessen the need to restrain me or isolate or seclude me from others:

I have these additional preferences for my mental health treatments:

7. Signature of Principle or Proxy or Other Legally Established Designee

By signing here, I indicate that I am mentally alert and competent and fully informed of the contents of this document, and that I understand the full impact of having made this advance directive for mental health, behavioral health, and stress management.

Signature _____ Date_____

Initials:_____   Date last updated_____

Page_____

8. Affirmation of Witness(es)

I affirm that the principle, or other designee, is personally known to me; that the principle, or other designee, signed or acknowledged his/her signature on this advance directive for mental health, behavioral health, and stress management in my presence; that the principle, or other designee, appears to be of sound mind and not under duress, fraud, or undue influence.

Witnessed by:

Witness: _____ Date_____

Witness: _____ Date_____

Initials:_____   Date last updated_____

Page_____